Movement and Child Development

Clinics in Developmental Medicine No. 55

Movement and Child Development

Edited by
KENNETH S. HOLT

1975

Spastics International Medical Publications

LONDON: William Heinemann Medical Books Ltd.

PHILADELPHIA: J. B. Lippincott Co.

ISBN 433 15180 3

© 1975 Spastics International Medical Publications

Printed in England at THE LAVENHAM PRESS LTD., Lavenham, Suffolk

Preface

To be able to move about at will, to be able to control our movements, to be able to use movement for our own purposes and benefits are valuable possessions. We realise the many advantages of movement only when we lose it, or when we see others who are immobile. It is such an all-pervasive attribute that it is taken for granted all too often, and it has not been subjected to scientific study as much as it might have been. Children make use of movement in many ways as they develop, and great efforts are expended in helping those children who are unable to move. It is reasonable, therefore, to give careful thought to all the inter-relationships of movement and child development.

The chapters of this volume cover a wide range. The early ones are concerned with the neurophysiology of movement. Then follow several papers which attempt to link the scientific theories with everyday practices. The final chapters which describe individual techniques are necessarily less precise than the earlier ones, but they represent the sensitive approaches of individuals who, through long experience, have created successful methods for helping children. The scientist studying basic mechanisms can learn from the perceptive observations of therapists, and should work with them to interpret the results of the research and its practical applications. In turn, therapists need to know more about child development and neurophysiology, and in gaining this knowledge and understanding, should find their practical work more rewarding for both themselves and the children. The distance between scientist and therapist is wide, but strands of communication between the extremes are being created, and it is hoped that this volume will contribute towards strengthening those strands into firm bonds.

For several years 'Action Research for the Crippled Child' supported research studies on this theme at The Wolfson Centre, London. As 1973 was the 21st Anniversary of this organisation, the occasion was acknowledged by holding a two-day symposium on the subject of 'Movement and Child Development'. The papers presented at that symposium, and three additional papers by Ann Harrison, have been arranged and edited to constitute the present publication. It is hoped that this subject will prove to be of interest to many readers and that this book will stimulate further research.

K. S. Holt

Contributors

MISS PRISCILLA BARCLAY
Senior Occupational Therapist (Music Therapy), St. Lawrence's Hospital, Caterham, Surrey, England.

MISS R. BARNITT
Occupational Therapist, Queen Elizabeth Hospital for Children, Hackney Road, London E2, England.

MISS H. LORNA BRAND
Physiotherapist, The Wolfson Centre, Institute of Child Health, Mecklenburgh Square, London WC2, England.

MR. A. BROWN
Lecturer, Physical Education Centre, University of Newcastle upon Tyne, England.

PROFESSOR KEVIN CONNOLLY
Department of Psychology, University of Sheffield, Sheffield S10 2TN, England.

MISS N. R. FINNIE
Deputy Director, Child Development Centre, Charing Cross Hospital, Fulham Palace Road, London W6, England.

MISS M. GILBERTSON
Superintendent Physiotherapist, The Hospital for Sick Children, Great Ormond Street, London WC1, England.

MISS ANN HARRISON
Motor Development Research Unit, Department of Psychology, University of Sheffield, Sheffield S10 2TN, England.

MR. G. J. HIGGON
Headmaster, Martindale School, Hounslow, Middlesex, England.

DR. K. S. HOLT
Director, The Wolfson Centre, Institute of Child Health, Mecklenburgh Square, London WC1, England.

MRS. MOYA E. HORTON
Physiotherapist, formerly at The Wolfson Centre, Mecklenburgh Square, London WC1, England.

MISS SOPHIE LEVITT
Physiotherapist, The Wolfson Centre, formerly Director of Studies, Centre for Spastic Children, Cheyne Walk, London SW3, England.

DR. M. J. MACCULLOCH
Senior Lecturer, Department of Psychiatry, Royal Infirmary, Liverpool 3, England.

MISS J. MCGUINNESS
Choreologist, Institute of Choreology, 4 Margarvine Gardens, London W6, England.

PROFESSOR P. ROSENBAUM
Department of Paediatrics, Chedoke-McMaster Centre, Sanatorium Road, P.O. Box 590, Hamilton, Ontario, Canada.

DR. LEWIS ROSENBLOOM
Consultant Paediatrician, Alder Hey Children's Hospital, Eaton Road, Liverpool 12, England.

MRS. VERONICA SHERBORNE
Lecturer in Movement, Redland College, Bristol, England.

DR. BARRY WYKE
Director, The Neurological Laboratory, The Royal College of Surgeons, Lincoln's Inn Fields, London WC2, England.

Contents

THE IMPORTANCE OF MOVEMENT FOR CHILD DEVELOPMENT

THE DEVELOPMENT OF MOVEMENT AND MOTOR SKILLS

RECORDING CHILDREN'S MOVEMENTS

THERAPEUTIC AND EDUCATIONAL APPLICATIONS

THE IMPORTANCE OF MOVEMENT
FOR CHILD DEVELOPMENT

CHAPTER ONE

How and Why Children Move

K. S. HOLT

Introduction

Movement is a fundamental characteristic of all living things. The observation of movement is evidence of life. Simple organisms consisting of only a few cells show movement. The more complex organisms elaborate simple movements into complex physical skills. These features apply to human beings just as much as to other living things, and, as will be described in subsequent chapters, they develop many skills which they are able to use for their own purposes and advantages.

Human movement begins long before birth. Peiper (1963) refers to several reports of movements observed in fetuses of less than 2cm length and just a few weeks old. Later, fetal movements involve flexion and extension of the limbs and certain automatic movements such as swallowing. The frequency and strength of these movements often reflects the internal state of the fetus. Even at this early stage the neurological mechanisms for these movements appear to be well established. Wyke describes the evolution of neural activity from this early stage in Chapter 4.

At birth, babies' movements are usually symmetrical, and consist of alternating flexions and extensions. Their pattern, strength and frequency reflect the state of the infant. These movements are said to be purposeless in that they do not reach a specific result, but they probably play a part in building up muscle strength and in creating those neurological links which are used later on in the development of more complex actions.

From this stage there are three major developments. Two are concerned with the development of complex physical skills from simpler movements. Gravity exerts a strong influence upon movements, so postural control must be acquired, and chain reactions become important in the development of complex movements and the determination of the pattern of movements. The factors concerned with the development of physical skills are discussed by Connolly and Harrison in later chapters. The third major development is the infant's acquisition of an awareness of movements and an ability to control them.

Complex movements are used in various ways. These include survival, exercise and gratification, and purposeful intentions. Survival depends upon the maintenance of internal movements such as respiration and circulation of the blood, and upon an ability to adjust to the environment such as by searching for food and fleeing from hostile creatures. Purposeful movements are made either to increase the individual's awareness of his surroundings, to manipulate his environment, or to communicate. These aspects of movement are summarised in Fig. 1.

1

Gravity and the Early Development of Movements

Gravity cannot be seen. Consequently it is very easy to overlook the important influence of this strong force. To appreciate its strength one need only experience the forceful dropping backwards of the head of a child being raised to a sitting position who has not yet acquired head control. From birth onwards gravity affects all our movements. Movements made in the direction of gravity acquire additional impetus and those made against gravity are subdued. Many of the earliest activities of infants are concerned with achieving and holding stable postures against the influence of gravity. The normal progression of early neurological reflex activity is directed towards this aim. The attainment of such anti-gravity postures as holding up the head steadily, sitting up, and standing enables the infant to begin to use his eyes, ears, mouth and hands to find out about his surroundings. This is an important requirement of early biological development. Fig. 2 shows a child of four years of age who has not yet acquired the ability to hold up his head. This greatly restricts his opportunities for using his eyes and ears, and hence produces secondary deprivation of development and learning. Fig. 3 shows a child who *can* hold up his head steadily against gravity, but seldom does so because he is both deaf and blind as a result of maternal rubella, and with his double sensory disability there is little biological advantage in striving to get into anti-gravity postures.

Chain Reactions and the Development of Movements

Those neurological reflexes which produce an immediate and obvious response such as the Moro, grasp, and asymmetrical tonic neck reflexes, appear to be more familiar to therapists than the chain reactions. Yet the neurological chain reactions are essential for the development of movement sequences. An initial movement makes it easier for certain other movements to follow; for example, in the case of a prone-lying baby, turning of the head to one side encourages forward extension of the arm on the face side and flexion of the opposite leg. Various manoeuvres such as supporting the shoulder and applying pressure to the buttocks encourage those particular chain reactions which lead to swimming and crawling movements. The chain reactions which set the pattern for movements are accompanied by supporting reflexes which help to stabilise and maintain the various postures which are achieved. Peiper (1963) described these reactions as follows: 'the initial chain reflexes . . . and . . . all the ensuing reflexes and the postures dependent upon them follow strict laws; these bring the child through reflexes of which he is not conscious, into the exact position under the given conditions to maintain the equilibrium which would otherwise be lost.' Chain reaction movements occur automatically without the child's conscious intervention, and, indeed, any attempt to introduce conscious control of these reactions interferes with their natural easy responsiveness. Fig. 4, which is reproduced from Pikler (1972) shows several ways by which a child can get to the upright position. All these different actions are dependent upon chain reactions.

Some infants with neurological disorders show delay and abnormality of motor development as a result of interference with these chain reactions, and several methods of treatment have been devised to overcome the difficulties. For example, it is thought that repeatedly moving a child through the movement sequences he would

2

follow if the chain reactions were intact, will stimulate both the acquisition of these reactions and the development of the movements. It is also thought that various forms of stimulation can be used to strengthen the chain reactions and so facilitate the performance of a difficult movement.

These points will be discussed more fully in later papers. At this stage only two points will be made: firstly, that we need to know much more about chain reactions and the development of movements than we do at present; and secondly, that chain reactions, although important, constitute only one part of the total picture of movement development in the young child.

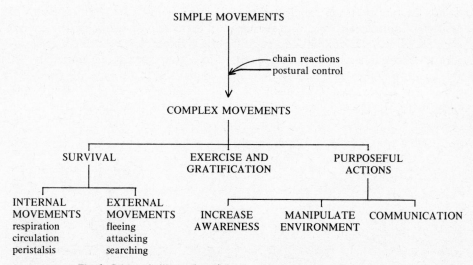

Fig. 1. Schematic illustration of the development and use of movements.

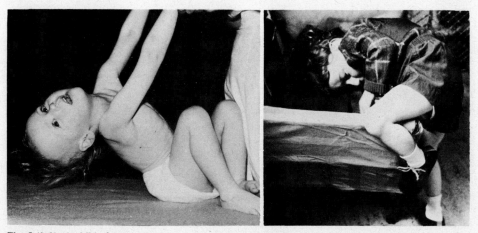

Fig. 2 (*left*). A child of four years who cannot hold up his head.

Fig. 3(*right*). A deaf and blind child who does not appreciate the advantages of being able to hold his head upright.

Sensorimotor Integration and the Control of Movements

By the time an individual has acquired anti-gravity control and a range of chain reaction movements, he is a stable mobile being. Further development occurs in humans as they learn how to modify and control movements, and how to put them to a wide variety of uses. The first step in this process consists of the development of sensorimotor integration. The brain must become aware of movements. The movement of a limb produces afferent stimuli to the central nervous system from joints, tendons, muscles, and skin, and these stimuli enable the brain to modify the strength, speed and frequency of the limb movements. In addition to the kinaesthetic stimuli, visual, auditory and tactile sensorimotor links develop to provide information which reveals the results of movements and in due course enables the brain to modify the position of movements, and to make use of movements for searching the environment. These sensorimotor links occur quite early in infant development. There is also good evidence (Jones 1974) that as the brain builds up concepts of movements it is able to anticipate, by initiating the movement fractionally in advance, the purpose for which it is being used. This ability enhances the effectiveness of sensorimotor integration. The importance of this integration is shown in Figures 5, 6 and 7.

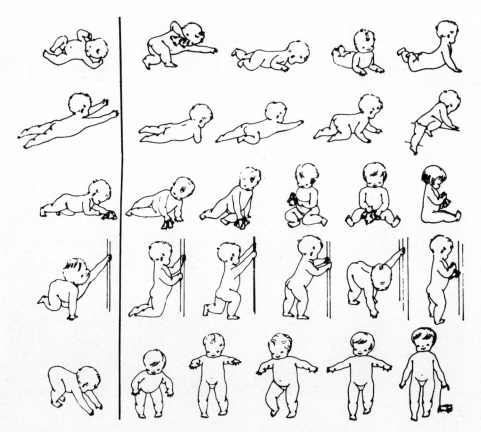

Fig. 4. Series of gross motor development on the basis of self-induced movements (from Pikler 1972).

4

The important step in the acquisition of control of movements is the development of awareness of the patterns of movements. Through the sensorimotor links already established, a child learns to observe movements, to analyse them into their component stages, and then to carry them out himself. This process is particularly well demonstrated in the evolution of children's ability to initiate gestures (Berges and Lezine 1965). The acquisition of an awareness of movement patterns is greatly helped by the development of a link between language and motor activity. Language skills enable a child to make more effective analyses of movement patterns, and to control the execution of motor acts by the use of verbal directions. It is a common experience to see and hear young children telling themselves what to do as they carry out a task, and many children enjoy skipping to jingles which reinforce and control the motor act. At least one form of treatment for motor-impaired children places great reliance upon the value of verbal reinforcement.

The Development of Motor Skills

Children perform many different motor acts. Those which are repeated frequently come to be performed increasingly skilfully. That is to say, they are carried out with progressively less and less thought and preparation, they are performed more quickly, precisely and smoothly, and the whole process involves less effort as the muscles are used more efficiently and effectively. There are many steps involved in the

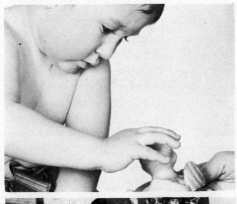

Fig. 5 (*left*). Visually-directed reaching and the development of hand-eye co-ordination.
Fig. 6 (*below left*). Head turning to locate the source of a sound—an auditory-motor link.
Fig. 7 (*below right*). Blind children using tactile exploration of their world.

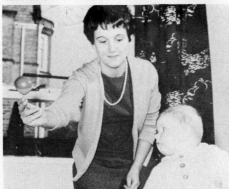

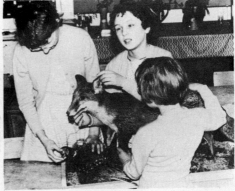

performance of skilled movements; for example, all the neurological chain reactions and the sensorimotor links must be intact. Hence many facets have to be analysed when motor skills are deficient, as in the case of a clumsy child. A better understanding of the importance of movement and child development will help considerably in the diagnosis and clinical management of disabled and clumsy children.

What is particularly remarkable about motor development in humans is the very wide range of motor skills they can develop as a result of their unique nervous system. All too often we accept without thinking such motor skills as typing, piano playing, dancing, and playing football. The wider aspects of these skills are mentioned in later chapters.

The Use of Movements

Humans are able to develop a wide range of movements. They are also able to put them to a wide variety of uses. There are the obvious basic biological purposes of movement, namely self preservation, exploring and gathering food. Humans, however, learn to use movement to control both themselves and their environment. Many are able to obtain pleasure from movements of some kind or other, whether this be a vigorous game of squash or a quiet walk through the countryside. Some use their abilities to control movements in order to promote their own physical and psychical status as, for example, in the practice of yoga.

Movement, then, is one of the principal means by which an individual controls his environment, both physical and emotional. On the physical side, the ability to move about, to explore, and to move objects, are obvious ways of demonstrating and exercising this control. It is, however, with respect to the development and control of the personal side of the environment that the great importance of movement is revealed. The impulsive movement towards, the hesitant step away, the twist of the head to seek or to avoid eye-to-eye contact, are all examples of how our movements reflect our emotional state. The child who runs to fling himself into his mother's arms, the one who plays hide-and-seek with his brothers, and the one who runs away from the school bully, are all making use of movement to express and to control personal relationships. Movements seems to be very important for a young child—for his pleasure, to enable him to learn about the world around him, and for him to develop normal emotional patterns.

The Effects of Impaired Movement

Clinical experiences with physically handicapped children led us to wonder about the effect of impairment of movement upon their development. This led us to realise the importance of movement in normal child development, and also led to two further steps. The first of these was to plan a developmental approach to the treatment of motor-handicapped children. This consists of three steps, as follows:
(1) analysis of the motor impairment according to a developmental pattern, and the planning of treatment to fit the developmental stage reached by the particular child;
(2) utilisation of those movement skills already possessed by the child for the purpose for which they were intended developmentally, if this is not occurring already;

6

(3) provision of those developmental experiences which the child is not receiving because of the lack of movement, in particular learning opportunities and emotional experiences.

The second of these steps led to a study of the value of developmental stimulation programmes for young handicapped children, which is described in later chapters.

In this symposium we will be studying the mechanism of movement, the developmental aspects of movements and lack of movement, and the results of remedial programmes. We begin by reviewing the neurological basis of movement.

Acknowledgements

Thanks are due to Gordon and Breach Science Publishers, Ltd. for permission to reproduce Fig. 4 from *Early Child Development and Care,* Vol. 1, p. 297.

REFERENCES

Berges, J., Lézine, I. (1965) *The Imitation of Gestures.* Clinics in Developmental Medicine, no. 18. London: Spastics International Medical Publications with Heinemann Medical.

Jones, B. (1974) 'The importance of memory traces of motor efferent discharges for learning skilled movements.' *Developmental Medicine and Child Neurology,* **16,** 620.

Peiper, A. (1963) *Cerebral Function in Infancy and Childhood.* Translation of 3rd German edition. New York: Consultants Bureau Enterprises Inc.

Pikler, E. (1972) 'Data on gross motor development of the infant.' *Early Child Development and Care,* **1,** 297.

CHAPTER TWO

The Consequences of Impaired Movement— A Hypothesis and Review

LEWIS ROSENBLOOM

When discussing the development of young children, it is customary to enumerate four different pathways along which progress is made, namely physical, intellectual, emotional and social. That there are close inter-relationships between all of these may be demonstrated readily, and advancement in one is almost invariably accompanied by progress in the others. Very many different factors influence the pathways of child development. The purpose of this paper is to review and discuss the contributions made by motor behaviour and to postulate that there may well be developmental consequences following impairment of movement.

Motor behaviour can be defined in a somewhat non-specific way as including children's *spontaneous physical activities*, both *gross*, for example those producing *mobility*, and *fine*, for example those producing *manipulative activities*. Evidence is available of the part that behaviour of this sort plays in fostering the development of physical skills, in contributing to perceptual, visuo-motor and language development, and in promoting normal emotional and social growth. Motor activity is also important as an integrating mechanism for linking together developmental progress in the four different pathways at any one period of time.

Prior to discussing these points in more detail, and also their therapeutic implications, one additional consideration merits mention. This concerns the existence of a feed-back mechanism whereby not only does a child's motor activity influence his ongoing development, but also the state of developmental maturity so reached in turn allows progressively more complex kinds of motor behaviour to be exhibited, and these then further influence his development.

Integrative Function

Returning now to a consideration of how motor behaviour acts as a linking and integrating mechanism in development, some examples can be given to demonstrate this. Consider first a baby about six months old who is just becoming able to sit. This particular motor activity as well as being a developmental stage in its own right also correlates temporally with the development of accurate reaching forwards and ability to grasp objects. Simultaneously, maturation of his visual behaviour enables the infant to fixate these same objects at six to twelve inches from his eyes for long enough periods to reach out for them. If we add to all this the fact that the erect position also now enables him to accurately localise the sources of sounds, then we can appreciate the dislocation to developmental integration that could occur if the infant's sitting were delayed.

Again, the motor behaviour of the three-year-old might be considered in relationship to his development overall. By the age of three, children are not only fully mobile but they can also use this mobility in activities such as climbing or riding a tricycle. This same mobility is also utilised in other activities for which the child is now sufficiently mature. These range from joining in play with other children, where there is for the first time the beginning of an understanding of sharing turns and playthings, to allowing the child the independence of going alone to the bathroom to wash his hands. In this way it is easy to see that inappropriate immobility in children of this age can readily lead to limitation of play opportunities and lack of independence.

All this is evidence of the inter-relationships between the different developmental pathways. Equally good cases can be made out for the significance of vision or language as mechanisms for integrating a child's progress towards maturity. The effect, however, of regarding motor behaviour in this way is to stress the importance of identifying children with motor handicaps and to increase awareness of the effects that these handicaps may have on over-all development.

Physical Development and Motor Skills

It is appropriate now to consider in more detail the varieties of motor behaviour that are significant and also the mechanisms by which they exert their influence. This is best done by discussing a number of observational and experimental studies, and first the relationship between motor behaviour and physical development may be examined.

Many stages of physical development are seen as a direct consequence of neurological maturation only. There is abundant evidence, for example, that in normal children the achievement of such basic abilities as sitting, standing or walking is determined primarily by this maturation, and that their emergence can neither be hastened by practice nor retarded by lack of it. What is important however, is that once the necessary neurological maturation has occurred, if the opportunity to practise these abilities is not given, then their further development and refinement will be retarded. This can be exemplified by considering the acquisition of skill in movement. Skill may be defined as the appropriate use of movement, and the appropriate use of exertion, space, control and speed, together with consistency of performance. It would appear that a skilful performance in a manipulative task such as pouring water into a receiver is seen only when there has been an opportunity to practice using the hands freely, once the necessary basic movements have appeared as a result of maturation. Certainly this was so in a group of children with spina bifida who were studied by a colleague and myself.* These children had had to use their ostensibly normal hands for support with walking aids or for manoeuvring their wheelchairs rather than in conventional manual exploration. It was found that their degree of manipulative skill was comparatively depressed and the most likely explanation for this is the specific decrease they had suffered in their manipulative

*Subsequent observations of children with limb deficiencies support these views. This information will be published in due course.

9

learning opportunities. Similar examples can be quoted for gross motor activities. Indeed one of the rôles of the physiotherapist in the nursery situation should be to promote increased skill in movement in young handicapped children, and this can be directly compared to the physical educationist's rôle in the education of both normal and handicapped children in school.

Perceptual, Visuo-motor and Language Development
The relationship between movement and aspects of intellectual development has been studied by numerous workers, of whom Richard Held has made perhaps the most significant contributions. Essentially his thesis (Held 1965) is that active movement, whether of the body as a whole or of individual limbs, is important for normal perceptual and visuo-motor development, and that this cannot be substituted either by passive movement or by no movement at all. Evidence is adduced for this hypothesis from work which he and his colleagues have done with kittens and human adult subjects. Thus in one experiment they devised a method by which the gross movements of a kitten moving actively were transmitted to a litter mate being passively carried in a harness. Both animals, one active, the other passive, moved around the same area, thereby obtaining the same visual stimulation. After some thirty hours of such experience it was shown that the active member of each pair showed normal behaviour on a range of visually-guided tasks such as accurate placing movements of the limbs, while the passively moved kitten failed to show this behaviour.

Other studies by the same workers have demonstrated that it is important for a kitten or monkey to view its own actively moving limbs if it is to make accurate visual placing responses, while so far as human adults are concerned, they have shown that if visual impulses are distorted with prisms, subjects under test will accomplish spatial tasks poorly, but can compensate somewhat for this poor performance if they are allowed to actively move either their whole body or one of their limbs, depending on what the particular task is.

Some work has also been done with human babies. This has shown that if active movements of the arms and hands are encouraged in the first few months of life (by providing brightly coloured, three-dimensional targets for the infants to aim at), the development of visual explorative behaviour and visually-directed reaching are accelerated.

Another interesting study is that of Denner and Cashdan (1967). They showed that children recall solid shapes better after handling them than when they had merely seen them. When the shapes were enclosed in perspex spheres however, so that the shape itself could not be manipulated although the perspex could, the children could remember the shapes just as well as when they were actually handled. This again would suggest that the amount of activity exerted is the crucial factor in the children's learning.

Thus the general conclusion is that motor activity has a wider significance for development than might at first be appreciated, particularly insofar as aspects of intellectual growth are concerned. Indeed, Jane Abercrombie (1968) said that limitation of an individual's capacity to exhibit active movement is likely to retard his

10

perceptual development generally and in this way limit his over-all intellectual ability. Abercrombie has also offered a very specific illustration of this concept as it affects children with cerebral palsy. It is well established that these children frequently have abnormalities of conjugate movements of their eyes, and it is theoretically possible to correlate this with the fact that many also have disorders of visuo-motor and visuo-perceptual functioning. In other words, there is here a possibility of a cause-and-effect relationship, with the movement abnormality producing the intellectual disorder.

Language learning is another aspect of development whose relationship to movement has recently been studied (Cashdan 1969). Most of this work has been done with children of subnormal intelligence, and it has been found that the initiation of language learning is facilitated if children are instructed and encouraged to speak and make relevant movements and gestures at the same time. In his review Cashdan pointed out how some workers have used movement very specifically in relating individual sounds and symbols to a system of gestural movements, while others have used the association between movement and language more generally by promoting a wide range of what are considered to be enriching motor experiences for the children in their programmes.

Emotional and Social Development

The contribution of motor behaviour to emotional and social development is another aspect of this subject that merits discussion. Unfortunately, although a great deal is known about the stages of emotional and social progress that children pass through on the way to maturity, acceptable and useful norms for assessing such things as personality and emotional status are not generally available. This obviously makes for difficulties should, for example, the relationship between some features of motor behaviour to a child's developing personality be the subject of a projected study. Knowledge and information has therefore had to come indirectly, and, as it were, in reverse, by examining the social and emotional disorders of children who have abnormal motor behaviour due to physical handicaps, and here at least, there is no shortage of information.

The frustration, dependence, and lack of social interaction that the child with cerebral palsy suffers are well known. Prevalence studies of the incidence of emotional disturbance have given figures of 40 per cent or more in these children and this is much greater than in the general child population. Most recently, in a study from the Isle of Wight (Graham and Rutter 1968) it has been shown that the incidence of psychiatric disorder in ten- and eleven-year-olds is 11.5 per cent in children with a physical handicap without brain involvement, as compared with 6.8 per cent of normal children and over 34 per cent in physically handicapped children who do have evidence of brain damage. These figures can be taken to suggest that specific motor difficulties are significantly related to psychiatric disorder, and that their effect is compounded when there is accompanying brain dysfunction.

As far as clinical features are concerned, it is uncertain as to whether any particular varieties of emotional disorder are seen more frequently in cerebral palsy compared with normal children or those with other developmental disorders.

However, certainly in adolescence, the increasing awareness of physical inadequacy in many individuals can lead to severe reactions such as hostility to parents, siblings and friends, and a sensitivity to kindness which they interpret as being hypocritical. Again, although there are many ill-founded statements in the literature on the personality characteristics of children who are physically handicapped, there is little that has been definitely established. One factor that may well repay further investigation however, is the lack of independence and initiative seen in many physically handicapped school-leavers, and it is possibly worthwhile to attempt to relate this to their parents and the parents' reactions to the children's relative immobility.

The conclusions that can be drawn then are that, just as children are influenced physically and intellectually by their motor behaviour, so also is their emotional and social development. And while it is certainly true that other factors such as associated mental subnormality do contribute to emotional disorders in physically handicapped children, their motor difficulties in themselves play a large part in the frequent failures of adjustment that are seen.

Therapeutic Implications

Given the existence of an extensive relationship between motor behaviour and development, it is perhaps as well to examine briefly the implications of this from a therapeutic viewpoint. One way to do this is by putting forward for examination a hypothesis that, for the satisfactory development of individual children, a normal spectrum of motor experiences is needed. What this hypothesis implies is the possibility of identifying those features of motor behaviour in children of different ages that are significant to their development. Appropriate and extensive study of normal children would be necessary for this, and the indices of measurement to be used might be in both physiological and behavioural terms. Thus, for certain physical skills, analysis of exertion, space, speed and control of movement is required; for perceptual development, analysis of the correct forms of active movement is needed; study of gestures has to be related to language development, and accomplishment of goals to be related to emotional development. In this way, the normal child's vocabulary of movement can be examined in detail, and, what is more important, what he is gaining from each section of this vocabulary may be ascertained. If this can all be done, a basis would then be established for the rational application of this hypothesis to children with motor disorders. Following evaluation of the motor behaviour and over-all development of individual handicapped children, it would be possible to provide a substitute programme of motor experiences. One essential in the compilation of such programmes is the knowledge of what children actually learn from different patterns of movement, so that similar learning opportunities might be provided from movement patterns that handicapped children are more able to execute.

Obviously, such programmes of substitute motor experiences would need to be incorporated into the total management either of individuals or of groups of physically handicapped children, and it must be stressed that they would be aimed at promoting over-all development, rather than acting only on whatever specific physical difficulties the children might have, although these latter cannot of course be ignored.

Much more work needs to be done if there is to be further definition of what has to be termed here the normal spectrum of motor experiences and its therapeutic applications. However the point of discussing it at this stage is to emphasize that not only is it impossible to isolate motor behaviour from child development as a whole, but also that there are practical implications in the study of motor behaviour for those who are concerned with the management of handicapped children.

REFERENCES

Abercrombie, M. L. J. (1968) 'Some notes on spatial disability: movement, intelligence quotient and attentiveness.' *Developmental Medicine and Child Neurology,* **10,** 206.
Cashdan, A. (1969) 'The role of movement in language learning.' *In* Wolff, P., Mac Keith, R. (Eds.) *Planning for Better Learning,* Clinics in Developmental Medicine, no. 33. London: Spastics International Medical Publications with Heinemann Medical.
Denner, B., Cashdan, S. (1967) 'Sensory processing and the recognition of forms in nursery-school children.' *British Journal of Psychology,* **58,** 101.
Graham, P., Rutter, M. (1968) 'Organic brain dysfunction and child psychiatric disorder.' *British Medical Journal,* **iii,** 695.
Held, R. (1965) 'Plasticity in sensory-motor systems.' *Scientific American,* **213**(5), 84.

CHAPTER THREE

Movement Disturbances:
Patterns of Overactivity and
Behaviour Disturbances in Children

D. SHAFFER

Overactive behaviour was described in brain-injured children by Still as long ago as 1902. In 1947 Strauss and Lehtinen published their monograph on the education of the brain-injured child. In this they elevated the status of overactive behaviour to that of a pathognomonic clinical sign, indicative of underlying brain damage. There has followed a seemingly endless series of papers describing overactivity in children with a history of premature birth (Drillien 1965), perinatal abnormalities (Pasamanick and Knobloch 1960), cerebral palsy (Ingram 1956), temporal lobe epilepsy (Ounsted *et al.* 1966) *etc., etc.* These studies have all been based on selected clinical populations, but most importantly, they have failed either to define overactivity (except in terms of subjective judgements), or to compare the children thus labelled with nonbrain-injured psychiatric controls.

What started as a behavioural description has almost imperceptibly become a nosological entity labelled the *hyperkinetic,* or *hyperactivity* syndrome. This carries with it implications of an organic aetiology, responsiveness to treatment with amphetamine-like stimulants and an unfavourable long-term prognosis.

The popularity of this diagnosis amongst child psychiatrists can be gauged from clinical surveys. In 1956, Patterson indicated that the hyperkinetic syndrome had become one of the most widely applied diagnoses in child psychiatric practice. More recently, Greenberg and Lipmann (1971) published a survey carried out amongst paediatricians and child psychiatrists in Washington, D.C. More than 40 per cent of the patients seen by the child psychiatrists had been given a diagnosis of hyperkinetic syndrome and more than 70 per cent of these had received treatment with stimulant drugs. A similar study in the Chicago area (Steven *et al.* 1973) indicated practice of the same order. Projecting from the survey findings, it was estimated that no fewer than 5 per cent of the Chicago school population would be diagnosed as suffering from the hyperactivity syndrome.

Acceptance of the concept has also been apparent in the ever-increasing volume of papers dealing with the effects of different forms of treatment on children with hyperactivity and studies describing their biological correlates and their prognosis.

The enthusiastic use of the concept of hyperactivity as a syndrome raises several problems. First, it is not a diagnosis which can be made with any degree of reliability. Kenny and colleagues (1971) arranged for 100 consecutive children diagnosed as 'hyperactive' to be rated by at least three independent observers. Agreement between all three was only obtained in 13 per cent of the referrals and 58 per cent of the children were not considered to be hyperactive by any one of the different raters. Given the frequency with which children are judged to be overactive by parents and teachers, this is not all that surprising. For example, Lapouse and Monk (1958), in their epidemiological study of a total population of 6 to 12-year-olds noted that more than 50 per cent of mothers considered their sons to be overactive. Similarly on the Isle of Wight, Rutter and his colleagues (1970) found that 35 per cent of boys in the general population were rated by their parents as being abnormally restless, 36 per cent of all boys were rated by their teachers as having poor concentration, and 16 per cent as being restless.

The second cause for concern about the increasing frequency with which this diagnosis is being used in a clinical setting lies in the contrast with its frequency in epidemiologically based studies. As mentioned above, many clinics seem to be making this diagnosis more frequently than any other in their psychiatric practice. Yet on the Isle of Wight only 1.6 per cent of psychiatrically disturbed children were judged to be suffering from the hyperactivity syndrome.

It would appear that many clinicians and perhaps teachers are confusing apparent overactivity in children with conduct or learning disorders with an allegedly distinct nosological entity. The evidence for this is best prefaced by a brief introduction into what we do know about the characteristics of children with a conduct disorder syndrome, and what are alleged to be the characteristics of children with the hyperactivity syndrome.

The existence of the conduct disorder syndrome as a coherent entity has been validated by a number of studies which have factor-analysed the presenting behaviours of a variety of groups of disturbed children presenting in different settings (Peterson 1961, Achenbach 1966). When this statistical procedure is carried out it will be noted that most disturbed children consistently fall into one of three major categories, *i.e.* a category in which antisocial symptoms predominate which is usually called the *conduct disorder, syndrome,* a category in which emotional symptoms, such as worrying, anxiety, depression *etc.* predominate and usually known as *neurotic disorder* or *emotional disorder* of childhood, and a third category in which children show a mixture of both antisocial and emotional behaviours. It is of interest that in terms of their antecedents and prognosis, this third mixed group most resembles the pure antisocial group. The characteristics of the children in the conduct and the mixed conduct groups have been defined consistently in numerous studies (Robins 1966, Rutter *et al.* 1970).

Children with antisocial disturbance are more likely to be boys, and tend to come from large families and broken or unhappy homes. There is a high rate of sociopathy in their parents and they have a high rate of learning disorders. The prognosis for these children is poor, many of them going on to develop sociopathic disorders in later life. Children with the hyperactivity syndrome are usually described as being overactive, having difficulty concentrating, having an impulsive response tempo, showing negativistic or antisocial behaviour and learning difficulties (Eisenberg 1957, Clements 1966). The syndrome is said to be commoner in boys.

Antisocial behaviour and learning disorders and a male predominance are therefore held to characterise both syndromes. Differentiation between the two disorders is usually held to rest upon the presence of overactivity, impulsivity and inattention in one group but not in the other (Stewart *et al.* 1970).

Strauss and Lehtinen's position, that hyperactivity is itself pathognomonic of CNS abnormality or dysfunction, is taking a long time to die, and it is commonly held that hyperactive children are more likely to show associated developmental delays or frank neurological abnormalities (Clements 1966), although there is little evidence to support this (Werry and Sprague 1970).

In an attempt to examine this problem experimentally, my colleagues and I (Shaffer *et al.* 1974) studied four groups of 5 to 7-year-old boys (see Table I).

TABLE I

Group 1: No conduct disorder.	No neurological disorder.
Group 2: Conduct disorder.	No neurological disorder.
Group 3: Conduct disorder.	Neurological disorder.
Group 4: No conduct disorder.	Neurological disorder.

The boys were categorised behaviourally by their score on a conduct disorder dimension of a well-tried behaviour disorder inventory (Quay and Peterson 1967), and neurologically by the presence or absence of gross neurological pathology, such as cerebral palsy or epilepsy. In addition, all boys in the neurologically abnormal group were screened for the usually acknowledged stigmata of the minimal brain dysfunction syndrome and those children with 'soft' sensorimotor signs or developmental EEG abnormalities were excluded. The children were studied in two settings for a period of ten minutes each. The first was a free-play setting. Motor activity was recorded quantitively by actometers (Schulman and Riesman 1959) attached to hands and legs. Activity shifts were recorded in a semi-automatic fashion. The boys were also studied in a highly structured setting when they were asked to sit on a cushion which recorded wriggling movement (Sprague and Toppe 1966) during the performance of an automated Continuous Attention Test. The experimental findings were subjected to analysis of variance to take account of differences in IQ and chronological age.

In the free-play setting the boys with a conduct disorder—irrespective of their neurological status—had mean actometer readings that were significantly higher than the boys without a conduct disorder ($F=6.1$, $p<.025$). Similarly, during the vigilance task, the boys with conduct disorders wriggled more than the psychiatrically normal children, although differences were not statistically significant. The conduct disordered boys also made more errors on the vigilance task, showed more activity shifts and were significantly more impulsive, when this was measured on Kagan's Memory for Familiar Figures Test (Kagan *et al.* 1964). When conduct status, IQ and age were taken into account, the presence of brain damage did not seem to have any significant effect on activity.

An implication of this study is that overactivity, inattention and impulsivity are non-specific features of the *conduct disorder syndrome,* that their presence does not warrant the conceptualisation of a new syndrome and that they are not necessarily linked to neurological dysfunction. A critical test of this hypothesis would involve the identification of a group of children suffering from a conduct disorder. Using

16

objective measurement techniques it should then be possible to identify high- and low-activity subgroups. Only if these groups differed, in terms of antecedent factors, or response to therapy or in prognosis, could it be held that the presence of high activity in a given situation is of any discriminatory value in children with a conduct disorder.

There is some evidence which suggests that this is unlikely to be the case. Cantwell (1972) examined the characteristics of parents of children whom he has labelled as being hyperactive. He noted a high rate of sociopathic personality disturbance in these parents. Sociopathy is of course also characteristic of the parents of children with conduct disorder (Robins 1966). Follow-up studies on children who had been diagnosed as being hyperactive (Menkes *et al.* 1967, Minde *et al.* 1972), have also been consistent in reporting a high incidence of antisocial behaviour during the follow-up period. Once again, a finding one would expect from studying children with a conduct disorder. Most studies on the hyperactive child record a high incidence of learning difficulties. However, Rutter *et al.* (1970) and others have reported a high incidence of learning disorder in conduct disturbed children as well. On the Isle of Wight the over-all incidence of reading backwardness was 4 per cent. However, this rose to 33 per cent amongst children with a conduct disorder.

In conclusion, it is proposed that the unjustified use of this concept, with its implications of a pervasive biologically based deviation, may blind the psychiatrist to the social and environmental determinants of the child's condition. There is much evidence to show that overactivity is situationally determined and is frequently a product of stress or inadequate motivation. Evidence linking hyperactivity and organic factors is at best tenuous and is in marked contrast to the importance that environmental factors have been shown to have in determining antisocial conduct in study after study.

REFERENCES

Achenbach, T. M. (1966) 'The classification of children's psychiatric symptoms, a factor analytic study.' *Psychological Monographs,* **80,** 6.
Cantwell, D. P. (1972) 'Psychiatric illness in the families of hyperactive children.' *Archives of General Psychiatry,* **27,** 414.
Clements, S. D. (1966) 'Minimal brain dysfunction in children.' *NINDS Monograph no. 3,* U.S.P.H.S. no. 1415, Washington, D.C.
Drillien, C. M. (1965) 'The effect of obstetrical hazard on the later development of the child.' *In* Gairdner, D. (Ed.) *Recent Advances in Paediatrics.* London: Churchill.
Eisenberg, L. (1957) 'Psychiatric implications of brain damage in children.' *Psychiatric Quarterly,* **31,** 72.
Greenberg, L., Lipmann, R. (1971) 'Pharmacotherapy of hyperactive children.' *Clinical Proceedings of the Children's Hospital, Washington,* **27,** 101.
Ingram, T. T. S. (1956) 'A characteristic form of overactive behaviour in brain damaged children.' *Journal of Medical Science,* **102,** 550.
Kagan, J., Rosman, B. L., Albert, J., Phillips, W. (1964) 'Information processing in the child: significance of analytic and reflective attitudes.' *Psychological Monographs,* **78,** 1.
Kenny, T. J., Clemmens, R. L., Hudson, B. W., Lentz, G. A., Cicci, R., Nair, P. (1971) 'Characteristics of children referred because of hyperactivity.' *Journal of Pediatrics,* **79,** 618.
Lapouse, R., Monk, M. A. (1958) 'An epidemiologic study of behavior characteristics in children.' *American Journal of Public Health,* **48,** 1134.

Menkes, M. M., Rowe, J. S., Menkes, J. H. (1967) 'A twenty-five year follow-up study on the hyperkinetic child with minimal brain dysfunction.' *Pediatrics*, **39**, 393.

Minde, K., Weiss, G., Mendelson, N. (1972) 'A five year follow-up study of 91 hyperactive school children.' *Journal of the American Academy of Child Psychiatry*, **11**, 595.

Ounsted, C., Lindsay, J., Norman, R. (1966) *Biological Factors in Temporal Lobe Epilepsy.* Clinics in Developmental Medicine, no. 22. London: Spastics International Medical Publications with Heinemann Medical.

Pasamanick, B., Knobloch, H. (1960) 'Brain damage and reproductive casualty.' *American Journal of Orthopsychiatry*, **30**, 298.

Patterson, C. (1956) 'A tentative approach to the classification of children's behaviour problems.' (Unpublished doctoral dissertation) University of Minnesota.

Peterson, G. R. (1961) 'Behaviour problems of middle childhood.' *Journal of Consulting Psychology*, **25**, 205.

Quay, H. C., Peterson, D. R. (1967) *Manual for the Behavior Problem Check List.* Champaign, Ill.: Children's Research Center, University of Illinois.

Robins, L. N. (1966) *Deviant Children Grown Up.* Baltimore: Williams and Wilkins.

Rutter, M., Tizard, J., Whitmore, K. (1970) *Education, Health and Behaviour.* New York: Wiley.

Schulman, J. L., Riesman, J. M. (1959) 'An objective measure of hyperactivity.' *American Journal of Mental Deficiency*, **64**, 455.

Shaffer, D., McNamara, N., Pincus, J. (1974) 'Controlled observations on patterns of activity, attention, and impulsivity in brain-damaged and psychiatrically disturbed boys.' *Psychological Medicine*, **4**, 4.

Sprague, R. L., Toppe, R. K. (1966) 'Relationship between activity level and delay in reinforcement in the retarded.' *Journal of Experimental and Child Psychology*, **3**, 390.

Steven, K. V., Sprague, R. L., Werry, J. S. (1973) 'Drug treatment of children in Chicago.' *In* Sprague, R. L. Werry, J. S. (Eds.) *Progress Report of Grant M.H. 18909.* Champaign Ill.: Children's Research Center, University of Illinois.

Stewart, M. A., Thach, B. T., Freidin, M. R. (1970) 'Accidental poisoning and the hyperactive child syndrome.' *Diseases of the Nervous System*, **31**, 403.

Still, G. F. (1902) 'Some abnormal psychical conditions in children.' *Lancet*, **i**, 1008, 1077, 1163.

Strauss, A. A., Lehtinen, L. E. (1947) *Psychopathology and Education of the Brain Injured Child.* New York: Grune and Stratton.

Werry, J. S., Sprague, R. L. (1970) 'Hyperactivity.' *In* Costello, C. G. (Ed.) *Symptoms of Psychopathology.* New York: Wiley.

THE DEVELOPMENT OF
MOVEMENT AND MOTOR SKILLS

CHAPTER FOUR

The Neurological Basis of Movement
—A Developmental Review

BARRY WYKE

Introduction: The Behavioural Significance of Movement

Although movements of parts of the body are effected by the synchronously co-ordinated contraction and relaxation of striated muscles—operating, for the most part, over joints—the stimulus to produce such movements, and the control mechanisms that regulate their execution and bring them to an appropriate stop, are neurological. In fact, in the circumstances of everyday life there are but two ways in which the brain may give overt display of its activity (Wyke 1959)—or, in other words, there are but two modes in which all human behaviour and misbehaviour may be expressed. The first of these—a *chemical* mode of expression, as it were—consists in changes in glandular secretion, as when we weep for sorrow or sweat with fear. The second is a *mechanical* mode of expression, and is manifest as changes of tension in visceral or striated muscles. These latter—the mechanical manifestations of the brain in action, with which we are here concerned—have a manifold significance that is not merely clinical; for in everyday life, the principal observable indices of nervous activity are presented by contraction and relaxation of striated muscles. Such phenomena thus provide the most tangible means of assessing the activity of the invisible living brain—so much so, in fact, that in the popular mind the presence or absence of movement is equated with the presence or absence of life itself.

It is with movements of his muscles that man ultimately establishes himself as a social organism, for his muscles are the instruments by which he communicates his thoughts and feelings to his fellows and by which they, in their turn, convey their mind to him (Wyke 1959). In short, it is by their motility that we can know the mind of others—a motility that involves principally the striated muscular apparatus of phonation, facial expression and limb movement. However, it is essential in the present context to point out that although mind expresses itself in motility, the execution of movements does not necessarily imply the operations of mind nor does their absence always signify the absence of mind—for nowhere is this more true than in consideration of the behavioural significance of the development of movements in the immature human organism, which topic provides the central theme of this chapter.

Nevertheless, it may be said that in mature man the cogitative functions of his brain ultimately fulfil themselves in the muscular activity of voluntary movement and postural adjustment. Thought and action become one, in so far as they are but two facets of the brain's activity—the first being internal and private and the second external and public. For whereas thought is a purely private and personal indication of his brain's functioning to the introspective man, action—manifest as speech and gestures, as well as in other movements and postural modifications—reveals to his fellows not only that he is thinking, but also (to a greater or lesser degree) the content and quality of his thought.

Furthermore, it is through its precisely controlled moving of the muscles of the body (especially those of the eyeballs, neck and limbs) that the brain is informed of the environment in which the body is located (Adrian 1928, Gooddy 1949, Wyke 1959, Sage 1971). Using the striated muscles as its tools, the brain probes and explores the external world by moving the body surfaces (armed as they are with an array of sensory receptors) through that world. In more esoteric modern parlance then, these sensory receptors continually 'scan' the world in which the body lives and moves and has its being, transmitting the resulting coded data through afferent nerves and tracts into the brain for analysis, storage or further action. Thus, muscular movements subserve for the brain functions that are not only expressive but are also apprehensive, for by its moving of the parts of the body the brain both learns of the world, and informs the world of what it has learnt (Wyke 1959). This aspect of the matter, too, is of moment to those concerned with the development of movement, for it must be appreciated that any impairment or restriction of a child's ability to move not only restricts his capacity to express his thoughts and feelings but also limits his capacity to inform himself of the world in which he is living, and thus automatically restricts the expansion of the range of the thoughts and feelings to be expressed that a normally-developing, mobile child experiences (Malpass 1960, Milner 1967, Zubek 1969, Connolly 1970, Cratty 1970, Sage 1971). This is one of the few aspects of its behaviour in which the brain resembles a computer, for with the brain, as with the computer, output depends on input; additionally with the brain, however, the on-going input is dependent upon the output in so far as the output is expressed in movements of the various receptor-equipped parts of the body.

Developmental Aspects of Neuromuscular Behaviour

In the light of these general (but nonetheless fundamental) considerations, I will now attempt to paint in, in broad strokes, a background of basic information relating to the developmental aspects of neuromuscular behaviour against which the subsequent chapters (dealing with particular aspects of normal and abnormal development) may be viewed.

The Emergence of Movement

The first (and most important) point to be made is that analysis of the neurological basis of movement in children cannot begin with the child (as it so often does in behavioural studies), but must begin with the fetus *in utero*, which is a highly mobile being long before it is born. In actual fact, a human organism is already about 100 weeks old (see Table I) before its neuromuscular mechanisms have matured to the point where it can stand and walk unaided.

During embryonic development, the striated muscle fibres—which are the source of the mechanical energy that produces movement (Needham 1960, Wyke 1969)—differentiate to a point, reached at five to six weeks (Gesell and Amatruda 1945, Hooker 1952, Boyd 1960, Murray 1960, Blechschmidt 1969, Hamilton and Mossman

20

TABLE I

Developmental Emergence of Neuromuscular Behaviour

Developmental period	Weeks of age from conception	Neuromuscular developmental phenomena
EMBRYONIC	5-6	Excitable muscle fibre differentiation. Innervation from alpha motoneurones.
	6-7	Motoneurone activation of motor units (through fine unmyelinated axons).
	7-8	Afferent neurones establish fine unmyelinated peripheral and central connexions (trigeminal system first).
	8	Oro-facial cutaneous mass reflexes elicitable. Ampullary cristae active.
FETAL	9-10	Mass 'spontaneous' movements of whole musculature. Moro reflex elicitable (from vestibular receptors).
	12	Muscle spindles differentiate. Movements of eyeballs. Generalized cervical reflexes. Palmar and plantar reflexes elicitable.
	14	Spinal grey nuclei differentiate. Fusimotor neurones active. Localized movements of lips, tongue (swallowing), head, trunk, limbs.
	16	Respiratory muscle movements (intercostals before diaphragm). First myelin lamellae in CNS (in cervical inter-segmental tracts and vestibular nerves)
	24	Myelin lamellae in spinal dorsal columns and medial longitudinal bundle. Commencing myelinization of cranial motor nerves, followed by afferents (vestibular first); and of reticulospinal, tectospinal and vestibulo-spinal tracts. Myelin lamellae in spinal nerves (motor before afferent).
	28	Facial mimetic muscle reflexes. Cervical reflexes regionally co-ordinated (Magnus and de Kleyn reflexes). Myelin lamellae in spinocerebellar and spinothalamic tracts.
	32	Vestibular reflex effects on eye and limb muscles.
	36	Myelin lamellae in cortical projection tracts, and in optic nerves.
BIRTH	36-37	
NEONATAL	38	Reflex walking, crawling and swimming movements elicitable.
	40	Ocular pursuit movements present. Voluntary control begins.
INFANCY	42	Reflex head extension in prone position.
	50	Visuo-motor reflex effects on neck, trunk and limb muscles. Positive supporting reflexes in arms.
	60	Head held up in supported sitting position.
	64	Sits unsupported. Exploratory creeping.
	68	Stands with support. Cerebral dominance emerging.
	70	Exploratory crawling. Positive supporting reflexes in legs.
	80	Walks with support.
	100	Stands and walks unaided.

1972) where they will respond to direct stimulation or to changes in plasma electrolyte concentration before the alpha motoneurones innervating them become capable of transmitting nerve impulses to them. This latter stage is reached during the seventh week of intra-uterine life (Cuajunco 1942, Barron 1953, Windle 1970, Hamilton and Mossman 1972) and occurs in respect of the cephalic and axial cervical muscles of the body before it happens in the limb and trunk muscles (Kingsbury 1924; Hooker 1952, 1954). In other words, then, the mechanical machinery that subserves movement in each part of the body is ready and able to operate before neurological controlling mechanisms are in a position to exercise any influence upon it; and such controlling mechanisms first become operative in relation to the musculature of the head and neck.

About one week after the contractility of the striated muscles in a particular part of the body is established, the alpha motoneurones in the related motoneurone pools become excitable, and segmentally-related afferent neurones differentiate* to establish peripheral extensions and central synaptic connexions (McKinniss 1936; Barron 1941, 1954; Mavrinskaia 1960; Windle 1970; Hamilton and Mossman 1972). The result is that generalized polysynaptic reflex muscular responses to mechanical tissue stimulation become elicitable during the eighth week of intra-uterine life (Hogg 1941; Gesell and Amatruda 1945; Hooker 1952, 1954; Humphrey and Hooker 1959; Bergström and Bergström 1963; Bergström 1969; Humphrey 1969c), first in respect of the oro-facial skin because trigeminal afferent and efferent neurones are the first of the peripheral nerve systems to mature to the point where they can transmit nerve impulses and thus to the point where they can exert reflexogenic influences on the striated musculature (Windle and Fitzgerald 1942; Humphrey 1952, 1954, 1969c; Hooker 1954; Bergström 1966; Darian-Smith 1966; Jacobs 1970). Furthermore, because of this developmental primacy of oro-facial mechanoreceptor afferents, the tissues of the mouth region remain a dominating source of afferent inputs to the developing brain until about three months after birth, when the visual input system takes over (Gesell and Amatruda 1945, Bosma 1967, Milner 1967, Bruner 1970). From about 14 weeks of intra-uterine age until this latter time, therefore, almost any mechanical stimulus to the upper part of the body leads to reflex flexion of the neck and arms, so that the hands are conveyed to the mouth; but prior to this (i.e. between the eighth and 14th weeks of intra-uterine life), oro-facial stimulation results in non-selective reflex head extension, lateral trunk flexion, and extension and abduction of the arms of the developing fetus, whilst cutaneous stimulation of the hand or foot produces generalized limb movements accompanied by digital flexion (Hogg 1941; Gesell and Amatruda 1945; Hooker 1952, 1954; Humphrey and Hooker 1959; Änggård et al. 1961; Bergström 1969; Humphrey 1969c).

So-called 'spontaneous' movements of the fetal body appear at about the ninth to 10th week of intra-uterine life but they remain generalized until about the 14th week, by which time more localized reflex movements of parts of the body have become apparent (Windle 1944, Gesell and Amatruda 1945, Hooker 1952, Bergström and

---

*Thus the number of neurones in the dorsal root ganglia of the upper cervical nerves more than trebles between the eighth and 13th weeks (McKinniss 1936).

Bergström 1963). Thus, the brain stem reflex systems that control eyeball movement begin to operate at about the 12th week (although they are not well established until the 24th week (Gesell and Amatruda 1945, Hooker 1952, Bergström 1969)), whilst the palmar digital and plantar toe reflexes (both of which are cutaneous mechanoreceptor reflex responses) become elicitable at the 11th to 12th weeks (Gesell and Amatruda 1945; Hooker 1952, 1954; Humphrey 1969c; Cratty 1970; Hamilton and Mossman 1972). Simultaneously, movements of the lips and tongue and swallowing movements begin to occur so that from now on the fetus continually swallows its surrounding amniotic fluid (Windle 1940; Gesell and Amatruda 1945; Hooker 1952, 1954; Peiper 1956; Humphrey 1969a, c).

Furthermore, at this time (i.e. during the 12th week) muscle spindles begin to differentiate in the individual striated muscles—again, first in the cephalic musculature—although they are not structurally and functionally mature until the 24th to 31st week (Hewer 1935; Cuajunco 1940; Mavrinskaia 1960, 1967; Bergström and Bergström 1963; Bowden 1963). Movements of the respiratory musculature become apparent between the 13th to 16th weeks, first in the intercostal muscles and later in the diaphragm, that from now on show increasingly marked variations in response to changes in the gas tensions (especially of carbon dioxide) in the mother's blood stream, although self-sustained reflex breathing is not possible until the 28th week (Gesell and Amatruda 1945, Hooker 1952, Bergström 1969). Reflex responses in the mimetic facial musculature and regionally-organized reflex responses to movements of the head on the neck also emerge at about the 28th week (Gesell and Amatruda 1945).

The vestibular receptor systems in the internal ear do not become reflexogenically fully active until the 32nd week, after which time a well-developed Moro reflex can be elicited (Schulte et al. 1969) until the child is between three and five months old. However, centripetal activity from the maturing ampullary cristae is detectable (as a feeble Moro reflex) as early as the eighth to ninth week of fetal age (Gesell and Amatruda 1945, Humphrey 1969b, Cratty 1970).

The Relevance of Myelinization

In view of the traditional behavioural emphasis that is always given to the progress of myelinization of nerve fibres in the developing nervous system (Langworthy 1933, Conel 1939, McGraw 1966, Milner 1967, Rorke and Riggs 1969, Connolly 1970, Hamilton and Mossman 1972), it may be appropriate to pause here to point out that the formation of myelin lamellae—which occurs as the result of the rotation of peripheral Schwann or central oligodendroglial cells around maturing nerve fibres (Wyke 1969)—has nothing to do with the assumption of transmission capacity by those fibres. It is merely a reflection of their maturational increase in diameter, and is thus epiphenomenally associated with an acceleration of their conduction velocity (Carpenter and Bergland 1957, Skoglund 1960, Wyke 1969). In fact, all functioning afferent and efferent nerve fibres and all central tract fibres in the developing nervous system are unmyelinated until the 16th week of intra-uterine life, when myelin lamellae begin to appear for the first time in relation to vestibular nerve fibres and in some of the intersegmental tract systems of the cervical spinal cord (Hamilton and Mossman 1972)—i.e. in the afferent fibres related to the mechanoreceptor systems

23

that are developing in the cervical apophyseal joints to subserve cervical arthrokinetic reflexes and (in later life) cervical kinaesthesis (Wyke 1966, Wyke and Molina 1972).

The entire fetal nervous system thus starts off as a small-diameter, unmyelinated, slowly-conducting system. Not until almost half of its intra-uterine lifetime has elapsed do some of the peripheral and central nerve fibre systems of the fetus increase above about 1.5μ to 2μ in diameter (when myelin lamellae begin to appear around them) and continue to increase in diameter thereafter, with parallel increases in their conduction velocity and peak impulse transmission frequency (Wyke 1969): in the pyramidal tract system, such changes do not even begin until about 10 months after birth (Lassek 1954, Humphrey 1960). Even in the adult nervous system, however, considerable afferent and efferent activity related to the regulation of movement continues to be subserved by small, unmyelinated (and thus slowly-conducting) fibres: for example, it is not widely appreciated that about 60 per cent of the fibres in the adult pyramidal tract remain less than 1.5μ in diameter, and are thus unmyelinated and slowly-conducting (Lassek 1954, Wyke 1959, Patton and Amassian 1960, Brodal 1969).

The importance of the increase in diameter of nerve fibres (with the associated myelinization and acceleration of conduction velocity) that does occur during development lies in its correlation with the exponential increase in body size that is a feature of prenatal and postnatal growth (Hamilton and Mossman 1972). As the distance of the parts of the body from the neuraxis increases (and thus the distance of peripheral mechanoreceptors from the neuraxis, and of the neuraxis from the striated muscles), so does the diameter of the mechanoreceptor afferent and alpha (and fusimotor) efferent fibres. This is associated with a gradual increase in the conduction velocity of the enlarging nerve fibres (Schulte *et al.* 1969), so that the transmission time from peripheral mechanoreceptors to the central nervous system and from the central nervous system to the striated muscles remains relatively constant in spite of the enlargement of the body. This is why *reflex times* remain relatively constant during childhood development, whereas *voluntary performance times* (which depend upon the efficiency of cerebral processing in central synaptic systems (Craik 1959)) decrease with increasing age during childhood (Hodgkins 1963, Connolly 1970, Sage 1971).

The Relevance of Mechanoreceptor Maturation

It should also be noted that maturation of the corpuscular mechanoreceptors in the various tissues of the body—especially in the skin (Kenshalo 1968) and in the capsules of the synovial joints of the limbs and vertebral column (Hromada 1960; Poláček 1966; Wyke 1966, 1972)—is determined by the mechanical stresses to which the tissues are exposed (Poláček 1956, 1966; Cauna 1959; Hromada 1960; Sklenská 1969). Such maturation therefore occurs (with the exception of the muscle spindles) mainly after birth, especially when crawling and walking patterns of behaviour begin to develop.

Thus, the more active a fetus is in the later stages of pregnancy, and the more handling and mechanical stimulation it gets after birth, the more rapidly will its tissue mechanoreceptors mature and the more efficient will its mechanoreceptor

24

reflexes become (McGraw 1935, Malpass 1960, Walters 1965, Sage 1971). Therefore, from the point of view of behavioural neuromuscular development, there is a lot to be said for the old Victorian nannie's dictum that 'babies should be bounced'. Conversely, lack of neonatal mobility (or deliberate immobilization in swaddling clothes, as still occurs in some cultures) retards corpuscular mechanoreceptor development, and leads to atrophy of any already existing mechanoreceptors (Poláček 1956, 1966; Sklenská 1969). As the stimulus/response characteristics of corpuscular mechanoreceptors depend upon their structural development (Wyke 1966, Iggo and Muir 1969), it will thus be apparent that immobility of the whole or of a part of the body in early postnatal (or later) life is a serious impediment to subsequent acquisition of efficient mechanoreceptor reflex activity, and of voluntary activity based on kinaesthetic inputs provided from the tissue mechanoreceptors (Thompson and Melzack 1956, Dennis and Najarian 1957, Malpass 1960, Scott 1962, Held 1968, Zubek 1969).

The Reflex Basis of Early Neuromuscular Behaviour

If we now return to consideration of the emergence of fetal patterns of neuromuscular activity, it should be emphasized that from about the 12th week of intra-uterine life movements of the trunk and limb musculature of the fetus are primarily effected as reflex responses to changes in the position of the head on the neck (Kingsbury 1924, Gesell and Amatruda 1945, Gesell 1954, Hooker 1954, Humphrey 1969c). Such changes are brought about randomly *in utero* by the pressure changes in the mother's abdominal cavity that result from her aortic pulsations, her respiratory movements, the filling and emptying of her stomach and the filling and emptying of her urinary bladder.

These fetal movements at first occur as feeble reflex responses to changes in vestibular input as the fetal head position varies; but later, by about the 28th week of intra-uterine life and increasingly so thereafter, their more vigorous production depends upon afferent discharges from the mechanoreceptors that differentiate progressively in the capsules of the cervical apophyseal joints (Wyke 1966, Wyke and Molina 1972). Thus, by the time of birth, the cervical arthrokinetic and myotatic reflex systems have become the major regulators of trunk and limb movements (Cratty 1970, Wyke and Molina 1972). These are supplemented by the now rapid maturation of progressively differentiating cutaneous and other articular mechano-receptor reflexogenic systems that operate through the fusimotor neurone-muscle spindle loop system (Eldred *et al.* 1953, Granit 1970, Matthews 1972, Wyke and Molina 1972), the development of which begins as early as the 12th week of intra-uterine life. The vestibular system progressively becomes of less and less relative importance in regard to the reflex control of muscular activity—except for the neck and external ocular muscles (Magnus 1924, de Reuck and Knight 1967, Cratty 1970).

Not least for this reason, then, it is essential for students of infantile behaviour to appreciate that the overt neuromuscular activity of very young babies is entirely reflex, and thus is a function of the posture (involving particularly the position of the head on the neck) in which it is examined, so that the neuromuscular behaviour of the same baby in supine, prone and supported sitting positions is quite different. Later, however—*i.e.* by about 14 weeks after birth—visuo-motor reflexes, operating through the tectum of the midbrain and the tectospinal tracts, also become of major importance in influencing movements of the neck, trunk and limbs (Connolly 1970, Cratty 1970).

Cerebral Cortical Contributions to Neuromuscular Control

Until 12 to 14 weeks after birth, motor behaviour is primarily an expression of brain stem, cerebellar and intersegmental spinal reflex mechanisms, and does not depend significantly upon the operations of facilitatory and inhibitory cortical input or output systems (see Editor's note). Certainly, cortical afferent and efferent systems are present anatomically, and cortical neuronal differentiation has occurred long before this time (in fact, since about the 20th week of intra-uterine life (Conel 1939, Lassek 1954, Humphrey 1960, Marin-Padilla 1970, Hamilton and Mossman 1972), but because of the small diameter (and thus of the slow conduction velocity) of their constituent fibres, and the absence of dendrites in neonatal cortical neurones (De Crinis 1934), these cortical systems play little effective part in the control of movement at this stage (Hines and Boynton 1940, Hines 1942, Kennard and Fulton 1942, Terzuolo and Adey 1960, Bergström 1969).

In fact, not until about four weeks have elapsed after birth is there any evidence that cortical projection systems are implicated significantly in the control of neuromuscular behaviour, and then only in respect of movements of the neck and eyeballs (McGraw 1966, Connolly 1970, Cratty 1970). For this reason, the general motor behaviour of an anencephalic infant is little different from that of a normal infant until about three months of postnatal age (Gamper 1925, McGraw 1966, Wolff 1969); but from then on, the maturing afferent and efferent cortical projection systems assume increasing potency in facilitating and inhibiting motoneurone activity (Wyke 1959, Patton and Amassian 1960, Terzuolo and Adey 1960, Milner 1967, Phillips 1967, Bergström 1969, Granit 1970). This occurs first, and most powerfully, in response to visual and kinaesthetic inputs and later (and additionally) in response to acoustic stimulation (Gesell and Amatruda 1945, André-Thomas and Autgaerden 1963, McGraw 1966, Connolly 1970, Cratty 1970, Granit 1970, Sage 1971).

After three months of age, movements of the individual parts of the body gradually become more particularized as cortical control mechanisms—which regulate afferent inflow (Wyke 1960, 1969; Hernández-Peón 1969), as well as the efferent activity delivered to the muscles from their motoneurone pools (Wyke 1959, Patton and Amassian 1960, Terzuolo and Adey 1960, Brodal 1969)—become increasingly efficient (partly as a result of the increasing fibre diameter of the afferent and efferent cortical tract systems) and are grafted onto the pre-established background of the complex of reflexogenic systems that have already been mentioned (Robinson 1969).

Finally, it should be noted that although cerebral dominance of motor control of the muscles of the right and left sides of the body begins to emerge at about six to eight months of postnatal age, it is not well established until the child is between 18 and 24 months old (Lippman 1927, Gesell and Ames 1947, Cohen 1966)—and in some children, not until their fifth year (Cratty 1970, Sage 1971).

Maturation of Neuromuscular Control Systems

Thus far in this account, I have tried to eschew abstract philosophical speculation (with which this field of study is only too replete) in favour of a factual summary—as far as is possible with the limited range of data at our disposal—of the processes by which neuromuscular activity gradually emerges in the developing human organism in the first 12 months of its biological existence (see Table I for details). Other chapters in this book will describe and analyse the behavioural events that occur in the infant after this period; but I want it to be clearly understood at the outset that the development of neuromuscular behaviour in the growing child is merely the temporal extension of a complex series of neurological processes that are genetically set in train long before the child sees the light of day.

I also want to emphasize that the neurological mechanisms that produce and control bodily movement throughout the first year of each individual's existence *are entirely reflex*, and as such involve changes in the patterns of activity of motor units that are determined by an increasingly varied array of afferent inputs fed into the neuraxis from the progressively differentiating and maturing receptor systems located in the various tissues of the body. To put it in crude terms, in the first year of its biological existence a human organism *does not move;* instead, it is *moved by* the galaxy of mechanical and chemical stimuli to which its central nervous system is continually exposed before, and immediately after, birth. This is not merely an esoteric academic point. On the contrary, I contend that it is fundamental to the whole theme of this book, concerned as it is with the problems of normal and abnormal development of neuromuscular behaviour in children; and if only this nettle could be firmly grasped, then a lot of the intellectual confusion that exists in this field of study might happily evaporate.

In the first year of its biological existence, then, a human organism is essentially a reflex machine, whose neuromuscular behaviour at any moment is an expression of the extent to which its various reflexogenic systems have differentiated and matured. Therefore, until it has attained about three months of age, a baby cannot be said to 'learn' anything of neuromuscular behaviour—for one cannot learn to *do* anything with one's reflexes: on the contrary, one's reflexes *do* things *to* one! Only when some three months have elapsed after birth can 'learning' processes be said to be involved in the emergence of further modifications in the patterns of a baby's neuromuscular behaviour, for only then do the slowly-maturing afferent and efferent projection systems of the cerebral cortex begin to exert significant modulating influences on motor unit activity (McGraw 1966, Milner 1967, Connolly 1970, Cratty 1970,). In this regard, as a neurologist I would insist that 'learning' is a cerebral function that involves the participation of the cerebral cortex, and that its effects must not be confused (as they so often are in neuromuscular behavioural studies) with the changing effects of adaptive reflex behaviour.

Immature reflex systems operate initially as simple 'on-line' systems, in which the parameters of the output are more or less direct functions of the reflexogenic input; and this appears to be to the case with the reflex reponses of the fetus in the first 10 to 12 weeks of its existence. Thereafter, the continuing process of neuro-muscular functional maturation involves, first, the development of increasingly elaborate facilitatory and inhibitory reflexogenic feed-back systems to motoneurone pools operated from the mechanoreceptors differentiating in the skin, joints, muscles

27

and tendons from about the 12th week onwards (Hagbarth 1952; Skoglund 1960*b*; Änggård *et al.* 1961; Melzack and Wall 1962, 1965; Wyke 1966; Gardner 1967; Kenshalo 1968; Schulte *et al.* 1969; Granit 1970; Matthews 1972); and second, the development (largely after birth) of central, presynaptic inhibitory filtering projections from the brain stem reticular system to the initial synaptic relays in the peripheral input systems (Wyke 1960, 1969; Hernández-Peón 1969). Some of these latter reticular projections—as the ultimate stage in the progressive sophistication of neuromuscular control systems—eventually become capable of voluntary modulations through the developmental maturation of corticoreticular projections, to the increasingly efficient use of which the term 'learning' can certainly be applied (Hernández-Peón and Hagbarth 1955, Galambos and Morgan 1960, Person 1960, Delafresnaye 1961, Brodal 1969, Wyke 1969). In this way, then, the developing individual gradually acquires feed-back (or servo-control) systems affecting his musculature. In these systems the onward flow of activity can be modulated up or down, initially by peripheral, and later by additional central regulatory mechanisms, so that reflex responses are no longer simple direct functions of stimulus intensity or frequency but are continuously being programmed by the prevailing 'set' of the built-in central input filtering systems. The refined control of these systems can certainly be (and normally is) 'learned', in conjunction with the emergence (also late after birth) of voluntary control of movements through the maturing corticobulbar and corticospinal projection systems.

Furthermore, it is relevant to re-emphasize that functional maturation of the central inhibitory filter systems seems to occur mainly after birth, and to develop with increasing effectiveness in the first three years of life, for the emergence of activity in these input filters apparently correlates with the increasing range and variability of afferent inputs to which the developing infant is exposed after birth—in contrast with the much more restricted afferent input into the neuraxis of an intra-uterine fetus floating freely in absolute darkness (albeit not in absolute silence) in a fluid medium of constant temperature. Nowadays, there is little doubt (at least, in the minds of many neurologists) that the nervous system reacts morphologically as well as functionally to environmental influences, within the limits set by its particular genetic inheritance (Hooker and Hare 1954, Galambos and Morgan 1960, Delafresnaye 1961, Bennett *et al.* 1964, Gaze 1970). This fact is witnessed, particularly in the present context, by the effects of changing mechanical stresses in tissues on the morphology (and thus on the response characteristics) of the receptors contained therein—as noted already in this chapter.

Finally, I would leave you with the thought that throughout the rest of his life *after* three months of postnatal age, an individual's control of his striated muscles remains dependent upon the background influence of the facilitatory and inhibitory reflexogenic mechanisms with which he was born, the relative importance of each component in which continues to be modified throughout life by increasing age and by environmental experience. Any so-called 'voluntary' movement at any age is therefore the ultimate expression, in the striated musculature, of the integrated effects (at the alpha motoneurone level) of a host of cortical and subcortical facilitatory and inhibitory influences, only a few of which are subject to the control of the

28

individual's will (Wyke 1959, 1969; Paillard 1960; Terzuolo and Adey 1960; Brodal 1969; Granit 1970)—which is why, incidentally, striated muscles should never be called 'voluntary' muscles. Last of all, I would beg those of you whose daily professional concern is with disorders of neuromuscular behaviour in children always to remember that a child's voluntary movements are only as accurate, co-ordinated, rapid and powerful as its reflexes and kinaesthetic inputs permit them to be (Lassek 1953, Twitchell 1954, Wyke 1959, Nathan and Sears 1960, Paillard 1960); and that disturbance of function in systems that are normally inhibitory is as disabling (or even more disabling) than disturbance of function in neurological systems that normally facilitate motoneurone activity, in respect of the acquisition and preservation of accurate control of movement.

Editor's note: This view will probably be challenged by some developmental neurologists because of increasing evidence of a number of activities by infants which almost certainly involve some cortical activity. Examples are: focussing by sucking (Bruner et al. 1966); head turning towards diffuse light (Goldie and Hopkins 1964); and responding to mother's voice (Bower 1966).

Bower, T. G. R. (1966) 'the visual world of infants.' *Scientific American,* **215,** (12), 80.
Bruner, J. S., Olver, R. R., Greenfield, P. M. (Eds.) (1966) *Studies in Cognitive Growth.* London: Wiley.
Goldie, L., Hopkins, I. J. (1964) 'Head turning towards diffuse light in the neurological examination of new-born infants.' *Brain,* **87,** 665.

REFERENCES

Adrian, E. D. (1928) *The Basis of Sensation. The Action of the Sense Organs.* London: Christophers.
André-Thomas, P., Autgaerden, S. (1963) *La Locomotion de la Vie Foetale à la Vie Post-natale.* Paris: Masson.
Änggard, L., Bergström, R. M., Bernhard, C. G. (1961) 'Analysis of prenatal spinal reflex activity in sheep.' *Acta Physiologica Scandinavica,* **53,** 128.
Barron, D. H. (1941) 'The functional development of some mammalian neuromuscular mechanisms.' *Biological Reviews,* **16,** 1.
——(1953) 'Some factors regulating the form and organization of the motoneurones of the spinal cord.' *In* Wholstenholme, G. E. W., Freeman, J. S., (General Eds.) Malcolm, J. L., Gray, J. A. B. (Consulting Eds.) *The Spinal Cord: Ciba Foundation Symposium.* London: Churchill, pp. 14-23.
—— (1954) 'The histogenesis of the spinal cord and the early development of behavior.' *Research Publications of the Association for Nervous and Mental Diseases,* **33,** 155.
Bennett, E. L., Diamond, M. C., Keech, D., Rosenzweig, M. R. (1964) 'Chemical and anatomical plasticity of brain.' *Science,* **146,** 610.
Bergström, L. (1966) 'Foetal development of mesencephalic motor functions in the guinea-pig.' *Acta Physiologica Scandinavica,* **68,** (suppl. 277), 22.
—— (1969) 'Electrical parameters of the brain during ontogeny.' *In* Robinson, R. J. (Ed.) *Brain and Early Behaviour Development in the Fetus and Infant.* C.A.S.D.S. Study Group on Brain Mechanisms of Early Behavioural Development. New York: Academic Press, pp. 15-37.
—— Bergström, R. M. (1963) 'Prenatal development of stretch reflex functions and brain stem activity in the human.' *Annales Chirurgiae et Gynaecologiae Fenniae,* **52,** (suppl. 117), 1.

Blechschmidt, E. (1969) *Die Entwicklung des menschlichen Nervensystems.* Göttingen: Hogrefe.

Bosma, J. F. (1967) 'Human infant oral function.' *In* Bosma, J. F. (Ed.) *Symposium on Oral Sensation and Perception.* Springfield, Ill.: C. C. Thomas, pp. 98-110.

Bowden, R. E. M. (1963) 'Muscle spindles in the human foetus.' *Acta Biologica, Szeged.,* **9,** 35.

Boyd, J. D. (1960) 'Development of striated muscle.' *In* Bourne, G. H. (Ed.) *Structure and Function of Muscle,* vol. I. New York: Academic Press, pp. 63-86.

Brodal, A. (1969) *Neurological Anatomy in Relation to Clinical Medicine,* 2nd ed. London: Oxford University Press.

Bruner, J. S. (1970) 'The growth and structure of skill.' *In* Connolly, K. (Ed.) *Mechanisms of Motor Skill Development. C.A.S.D.S. Study Group on Mechanisms of Motor Skill Development.* London and York: Academic Press, pp. 63-92.

Carpenter, F. G., Bergland, R. M. (1957) 'Excitation and conduction in immature nerve fibers of the developing chick.' *American Journal of Physiology,* **190,** 371.

Cauna, N. (1959) 'The mode of termination of sensory nerves and its significance.' *Journal of Comparative Neurology,* **113,** 169.

Cohen, A. I. (1966) 'Hand preference and developmental status of infants.' *Journal of Genetic Psychology,* **108,** 337.

Conel, J. L. (1939) *The Postnatal Development of the Human Cerebral Cortex. Vol. I. The Cortex of the Newborn.* Cambridge, Mass.: Harvard University Press.

Connolly, K. (Ed.) (1970) *Mechanisms of Motor Skill Development. C.A.S.D.S. Study Group on Mechanisms of Motor Skill Development.* London and New York: Academic Press.

Craik, K. J. W. (1969) 'Theory of the human operator in control systems. II. Man as example in a control system.' *In* Evans, C. R., Robinson, A. D. J. (Eds.) *Cybernetics.* London: Butterworths.

Cratty, B. J. (1970) *Perceptual and Motor Development in Infants and Children.* London: Macmillan.

Crinis, M. de (1934) *Aufbau und Abbau der Grosshirnleistungen und ihre anatomischen Grundlagen.* Berlin: Karger.

Cuajunco, F. (1940) 'Development of the neuro-muscular spindle in human fetuses.' *Contributions to Embryology,* **30,** 97.

—— (1942) 'Development of the human motor end plate.' *Contributions to Embryology,* **30,** 127.

Darian-Smith, I. (1966) 'Neural mechanisms of facial sensation.' *International Review of Neurobiology,* **9,** 301.

Delafresnaye, J. F. (Ed.) (1961) *Brain Mechanisms and Learning. A Symposium.* Oxford: Blackwell Scientific Publications.

Dennis, W., Najarian, P. (1957) 'Infant development under environmental handicap.' *Psychological Monographs,* **71,** no. 7, 1.

Eldred, E., Granit, R., Merton, P. A. (1953) 'Supraspinal control of the muscle spindles and its significance.' *Journal of Physiology,* **122,** 498.

Galambos, R., Morgan, C. T. (1960) 'The neural basis of learning.' *In* Field, J., Magoun, H. W., Hall, V. E. (Eds.) *Handbook of Physiology, section 1. Neurophysiology. Vol. III.* Washington: American Physiological Society, pp. 1471-1499.

Gamper, E. (1925) 'Bau und Leistungen eines menschlichen Mittelhirnwesens (Arhinencephalie mit Encephalocele) zugleich ein Beitrag zur Teratologie und Fasersystematik.' *Zeitschrift für die gesamte Neurologie und Psychiatrie,* **102,** 154.

Gardner, E. (1967) 'Spinal cord and brain stem pathways for afferents from joints.' *In* de Reuck, A. V. S., Knight, J. (Eds.) *Myotatic, Kinesthetic and Vestibular Mechanisms.* Ciba Foundation Symposium. Boston: Little, Brown, pp. 56-76.

Gaze, R. M. (1970) *The Formation of Nerve Connections: a Consideration of Neural Specificity Modulation and Comparable Phenomena.* London and New York: Academic Press.

Gesell, A. (1954) 'Behavior patterns of fetal-infant and child with evidences of innate growth patterns.' *Research Publications of the Association for Nervous and Mental Diseases,* **33,** 114.

—— Amatruda, C. S. (1945) *The Embryology of Behavior: The Beginnings of the Human Mind.* New York: Harper.

—— Ames, L. B. (1947) 'The development of handedness.' *Journal of Genetic Psychology,* **70,** 155.

Gooddy, W. (1949) 'Sensation and violition.' *Brain,* **72,** 312.

Granit, R. (1970) *The Basis of Motor Control.* London and New York: Academic Press.

Hagbarth, K.-E. (1952) 'Excitatory and inhibitory skin areas for flexor and extensor motoneurons.' *Acta Physiologica Scandinavica,* **26,** (Suppl. 94), 1.

Hamilton, W. J., Mossman, H. W. (1972) *Human Embryology: Prenatal Development of Form and Function.* 4th ed. Cambridge: Heffer.

Held, R. (1968) 'Plasticity in sensorimotor coordination.' *In* Freedman, S. J. (Ed.) *The Neuropsychology of Spatially Oriented Behavior.* Homewood, Ill.: Dorsey Press, pp. 57-62.

Hernández-Peón, R. (1969) 'A neurophysiological and evolutionary model of attention.' *In* Evans, C. R., Mulholland, T. B. (Eds.) *Attention in Neurophysiology.* London: Butterworths, pp. 417-432.

—— Hagbarth, K.-E. (1955) 'Interaction between afferent and cortically induced reticular responses.' *Journal of Neurophysiology,* **18,** 44.

Hewer, E. E. (1935) 'The development of nerve endings in the human foetus.' *Journal of Anatomy,* **69,** 369.

Hines, M. (1942) 'The development and regression of reflexes, postures and progression in the young macaque.' *Publications of the Carnegie Institute,* **541,** 153.

—— Boynton, E. P. (1940) 'The maturation of 'excitability' in the precentral gyrus of the young monkey (Macaca mulatta).' *Publications of the Carnegie Institute,* **518,** 309.

Hodgkins, J. (1963) 'Reaction time and speed of movement in males and females of various ages.' *Research Quarterly,* **34,** 335.

Hogg, I. D. (1941) 'Sensory nerves and associated structures in the skin of human fetuses of 8 to 14 weeks of menstrual age correlated with functional capability.' *Journal of Comparative Neurology,* **75,** 371.

Hooker, D. (1952) *The Prenatal Origin of Behavior.* Lawrence, Kansas: University of Kansas Press.

—— (1954) 'Early human fetal behavior with preliminary note on double simultaneous fetal stimulation.' *Research Publications of the Association for Nervous and Mental Disease,* **33,** 98.

—— Hare, C. C. (Eds.) (1954) *Genetics and the Inheritance of Integrated Nuerological and Psychiatric Patterns.* Baltimore: Williams and Wilkins.

Hromada, J. (1960) 'Beitrag zur Kenntnis der Entwicklung und der Variabilität der Lamellenkörperchen in der Gelenkkapsel und im periarticularen Gewebe beim menschlichen Fetus.' *Acta Anatomica,* **40,** 27.

Humphrey, T. (1952) 'The spinal tract of the trigeminal nerve in human embryos between 7½ and 8½ weeks of menstrual age and its relation to early fetal behavior.' *Journal of Comparative Neurology,* **97,** 143.

—— (1954) 'The trigeminal nerve in relation to early human fetal activity.' *Research Publications of the Association for Nervous and Mental Diseases,* **33,** 127.

—— (1960) 'The development of the pyramidal tract in human fetuses, correlated with cortical differentiation.' *In* Tower, D. B., Schadé, J. P. (Eds.) *Structure and Function of the Cerebral Cortex.* Amsterdam: Elsevier, pp. 94-103.

—— (1969*a*) 'The relation between human fetal mouth opening reflexes and closure of the palate.' *American Journal of Anatomy,* **125,** 317.

—— (1969*b*) 'Discussion'. *In* Robinson, R. J. (Ed.) *Brain and Early Behaviour Development in the Fetus and Infant. C.A.S.D.S. Study Group on Brain Mechanisms of Early Behavioural Development.* London and New York: Academic Press, pp. 40-41.

—— (1969*c*) 'Postnatal repetition of human prenatal activity sequences with some suggestions of their neuroanatomical basis. *In* Robinson, R. J. (Ed.) *Brain and Early Behaviour Development in the Fetus and Infant. C.A.S.D.S. Study Group on Brain Mechanisms of Early Behavioural Development.* London and New York: Academic Press, pp. 43-84.

—— Hooker, D. (1959) 'Double simultaneous stimulation of human fetuses and the anatomical patterns underlying the reflexes elicited.' *Journal of Comparative Neurology,* **112,** 75.

Iggo, A., Muir, A. R (1969) 'The structure and function of a slowly adapting touch corpuscle in hairy skin.' *Journal of Physiology,* **200,** 763.

Jacobs, M. J. (1970) 'The development of the human motor trigeminal complex and accessory facial nucleus and their topographic relations with the facial and abducens nuclei.' *Journal of Camparative Neurology,* **138,** 161.

Kennard, M. A., Fulton, J. F. (1942) 'Age and reorganization of central nervous system.' *Journal of Mt. Sinai Hospital,* **9,** 594.

Kenshalo, D. R. (Ed.) (1968) *The Skin Senses. Proceedings of the First International Symposium on the Skin Senses.* Springield, Ill.: C. C. Thomas.

Kingsbury, B. F. (1924) 'The significance of the so-called law of cephalo-caudal differential growth.' *Anatomical Record,* **27,** 305.

Langworthy, O. R. (1933) 'Development of behavior patterns and myelinization of the nervous system in the human fetus and infant.' *Contributions to Embryology,* **34,** 3.

Lassek, A. M. (1953) 'Inactivation of voluntary motor function following rhizotomy.' *Journal of Neuropathology and Experimental Neurology,* **12,** 83.

—— (1954) *The Pyramidal Tract.* Springfield, Ill.: C. C. Thomas.

Lippman, H. S. (1927) 'Certain behavior responses in early infancy.' *Journal of Genetic Psychology,* **34,** 424.

31

McGraw, M. B. (1935) *Growth. A Study of Johnny and Jimmy.* New York: Appleton-Century-Crofts.
—— (1966) *The Neuromuscular Maturation of the Human Infant. Revised ed.* New York: Hafner.
McKinniss, M. E. (1936) 'The number of ganglion cells in the dorsal root ganglia of the second and third cervical nerves of various ages.' *Anatomical Record,* **65,** 255.
Magnus, R. (1924) *Körperstellung; experimentall-physiologische Untersuchungen über die Einzelnen bei der Körperstellung in tätigkeit tretenden Reflexe, über ihr Zusammenwirken und ihre Störungen.* Berlin: Springer.
Malpass, L. F. (1960) Motor proficiency in institutionalized and non-institutionalized retarded and normal children.' *American Journal of Mental Deficiency,* **64,** 1012.
Marin-Padilla, M. (1970) 'Prenatal and early postnatal ontogenesis of the human motor cortex: a Golgi study. I. The sequential development of the cortical layer.' *Brain Research,* **23,** 167.
Matthews, P. B. C. (1972) *Mammalian Muscle Receptors and their Central Actions.* London: Arnold.
Mavrinskaia, L. F. (1960) 'On the relationship between the development of the nerve endings of the skeletal muscles and the appearance of movement activity in the human fetus.' *Arkhiv Anatomii,* **38,** 61.
—— (1967) 'Development of neuro-muscular spindles in man.' *Arkhiv Anatomii,* **53,** 42.
Melzack, R., Wall, P. D. (1962) 'On the nature of cutaneous sensory mechanisms.' *Brain,* **85,** 331.
—— (1965) 'Pain mechanisms: a new theory.' *Science,* **150,** 971.
Milner, E. (1967) *Human Neural and Behavioral Development.* Springfield, Ill.: C. C. Thomas.
Murray, M. M. (1960) 'Skeletal muscle tissue in culture.' *In* Bourne, G. H. (Ed.) *Structure and Function of Muscle, vol. I.* New York: Academic Press, pp. 111-136.
Nathan, P. W., Sears, T. A. (1960) 'Effects of posterior root section on the activity of some muscles in man.' *Journal of Neurology, Neurosurgery and Psychiatry,* **23,** 10.
Needham, D. H. (1960) 'Biochemistry of muscular action.' *In* Bourne, G. H. (Ed.) *Structure and Function of Muscle, vol. II.* New York: Academic Press, pp. 55-104.
Paillard, J. (1960) 'The patterning of skilled movements.' *In* Field, J., Magoun, H. W., Hall, V. E. (Eds.). *Handbook of Physiology. Section 1. Neurophysiology, vol. III.* Washington: American Physiological Society, pp. 1679-1708.
Patton, H. D., Amassian, V. E. (1960) 'The pyramidal tract: its excitation and functions.' *In* Field, J., Magoun, H. W., Hall, V. E. (Eds.) *Handbook of Physiology. Section 1. Neurophysiology,* vol. II. Washington: American Physiological Society, pp. 837-861.
Peiper, A. (1956) *Die Eigenart der kindlichen Hirntätigkeit.* Leipzig: Thieme.
Person, R. S. (1960) 'Studies of human movements when elaborating motor habits.' *In Proceedings of the Third International Conference on Medical Electronics, London.* Springfield, Ill.: C. C. Thomas, pp. 206-208.
Phillips, C. G. (1967) 'Corticomotoneuronal organization. Projection from the arm area of the baboon's motor cortex.' *Archives of Neurology,* **17,** 188.
Poláček, P. (1956) 'Morphological changes in the innervation of the joints in laboratory animals under experimental functional and pathological conditions.' *Acta Chirurgiae, Orthopaedicae et Traumatologiae Čechoslavaca,* **23,** 286.
—— (1966) *Receptors of the Joints. Their Structure, Variability and Classification.* Brno: Purkyné University Press.
Reuck, A. V. S. de, Knight, J. (Eds.) (1967) *Myotatic, Kinesthetic and Vestibular Mechanisms.* Ciba Foundation Symposium. Boston: Little, Brown.
Robinson, R. J. (Ed.) (1969) *Brain and Early Behaviour Development in the Fetus and Infant. C.A.S.D.S. Study Group on Brain Mechanisms of Early Behavioural Development.* London and New york: Academic Press.
Rorke, L. B., Riggs, H. E. (1969) *Myelination of the Brain in the Newborn.* Philadelphia: Lippincott.
Sage, G. H. (1971) *Introduction to Motor Behavior: A Neuropsychological Approach.* Reading, Mass.: Addison-Wesley.
Schulte, F. J., Linke, I., Michaelis, R., Nolte, R. (1969) 'Excitation, inhibition and impulse conduction in spinal motoneurones of preterm, term and small-for-dates newborn infants.' *In* Robinson, R. J. (Ed.) *Brain and Early Behaviour Development in the Fetus and Infant. C.A.S.D.S. Study Group on Brain Mechanisms of Early Behavioural Development.* New York: Academic Press, pp. 87-109.
Scott, J. P. (1962) 'Critical periods in behavioural development.' *Science,* **138,** 949.
Sklenská, A. (1969) Personal communication.
Skoglund, S. (1960*a*) 'The spingal transmission of proprioceptive reflexes and the postnatal development of conduction velocity in different hindlimb nerves in the kitten.' *Acta Physiologica Scandinavica,* **49,** 318.
—— (1960*b*) 'The activity of muscle receptors in the kitten.' *Acta Physiologica Scandinavica,* **50,** 203.

Terzuolo, C. A., Adey, W. R. (1960) 'Sensorimotor cortical activities.' *In* Field, J., Magoun, H. W., Hall, V. E. (Eds.) *Handbook of Physiology. Section 1. Neurophysiology, vol. II.* Washington: American Physiological Society, pp. 797-836

Thompson, W. R., Melzack, R. (1956) 'Early environment.' *Scientific American,* **194,** 38.

Twitchell, T. W. (1954) 'Sensory factors in purposive movement.' *Journal of Neurophysiology,* **17,** 239.

Walters, C. E. (1965) 'Prediction of post-natal development from foetal activity.' *Child Development,* **33,** 801.

Windle, W. F. (1940) *Physiology of the Fetus, Origin and Extent of Function in Prenatal Life.* Philadelphia: Saunders.

—— (1944) 'Genesis of somatic motor function in mammalian embryos: a synthesizing article.' *Physiological Zoology,* **17,** 247.

—— (1970) 'Development of neural elements in human embryos of four to seven weeks gestation.' *Experimental Neurology,* **28,** Suppl. 5 (II), 44.

—— Fitzgerald, J. E. (1942) 'Development of the human mesencephalic trigeminal root and related neurons.' *Journal of Comparative Neurology,* **77,** 597.

Wolff, P. H. (1969) 'Motor development and holotelencephaly.' *In* Robinson, R. J. (Ed.) *Brain and Early Behaviour Development in the Fetus and Infant. C.A.S.D.S. Study Group on Brain Mechanisms of Early Behavioural Development.* New York: Academic Press, pp. 139-162.

Wyke, B. D. (1959) 'The cortical control of movement.' *Epilepsia,* **1,** 4.

—— (1960) *Neurological Aspects of Hypnosis.* London: Dental and Medical Society for the Study of Hypnosis.

—— (1966) 'The neurology of joints.' *Annals of the Royal College of Surgeons of England,* **41,** 25.

—— (1969) *Principles of General Neurology. An Introduction to the Basic Principles of Medical and Surgical Neurology.* Amsterdam and London: Elsevier.

—— (1972) 'Articular neurology—a review.' *Physiotherapy,* **58,** 94.

—— Molina, F. (1972) 'Articula reflexology of the cervical spine.' *Proceedings of the Sixth International Congress of Physical Medicine. Barcelona,* p. 4.

Zubek, J. P. (Ed.) (1969) *Sensory Deprivation. Fifteen Years of Research.* New York: Appleton-Century-Crofts.

CHAPTER FIVE

Components of Neuromuscular Control

ANN HARRISON

A number of useful levels of analysis are available for describing motor control and motor skills. Within a cognitive framework, we can examine how well a person understands a task, how adequately he plans a movement and whether he appreciates and remedies any errors that he makes. In contrast, movements can be explained in purely mechanical terms. Forces are created as muscles contract and the movements which are observed reflect changes in the underlying pattern of contractile forces. Studying the physiological basis of motor control offers a guide to the functional complexity of the neuromuscular system. It indicates the large range of events which can affect movements and the many sources of information which may be used by a subject to judge his performance. It also provides a format for describing 'pathology', 'skill' and 'development' in terms of the physiological changes which characterise these. The usefulness of any one approach depends upon the question which is being asked.

This paper represents an attempt to understand how limb movements are achieved and to explain why spastic persons have difficulty in achieving good motor control. The problem is to assess the functional implications of those physiological abnormalities which are known to form the basis of the spastic syndrome. The approach which has been chosen is to use what is known of how neurologically normal individuals programme contractions, monitor neuromuscular activity and improve their motor control in order to infer the difficulties which face spastic individuals.

Skeletal Movements

Changes in posture and changes in limb orientation are achieved by the contraction of skeletal muscles. When antagonist muscles are present at a joint, the movement which is observed reflects the relative length of the agonist and antagonist muscles. Precise joint movements therefore require that activity in both these muscles is regulated accurately. Coactivation may be used to achieve better movement control, and activity in the antagonist provides a braking which can be used to regulate contractions and to bring fast contractions to a smooth stop.

An initial imbalance between the power of antagonist muscles may lead to joint deformities and movement abnormalities. Apparently weak muscles sometimes possess normal strength: the appearance of weakness stems from the fact that they are seen working in opposition to abnormally strong antagonists. Differences in muscle power tend to become increasingly more marked because the stronger muscle usually grows at a faster rate and because the weaker muscle may atrophy. As bone growth occurs, the joint deformity that results from muscle imbalance is accentuated (Sharrard 1974). When a joint becomes deformed, effective movement is even more difficult to achieve. Bone abnormalities and muscle abnormalities can each trigger the other, and it is therefore sometimes difficult to diagnose the cause of syndromes which involve both of these. This creates problems when the correct choice of therapy requires this distinction to be made.

Most limb movements involve activity in more than one set of muscles. Each contraction must be regulated so that the force it contributes increases and wanes appropriately. The correct movement will be achieved only if constituent contractions are activated in the correct temporal sequence and if potential sources of interference are controlled.

Muscular Contractions

Skeletal muscles are composed of bundles of *extrafusal* and *intrafusal* muscle fibres that lie parallel along the length of the muscle (Fig. 1). Sufficient activity in the *alpha efferent* pathway causes extrafusal fibres to contract and the muscle is seen to shorten. When a given alpha motoneuron fires, a fixed group of extrafusal fibres contracts fully. As more alpha motoneurons become active, the over-all length of the muscle decreases and the force generated by the contraction increases. A single alpha motoneuron and the fibres activated by it constitute a *motor unit*. The force produced when a single motor unit is fired defines the smallest step with which the contractile strength can be increased or decreased. The size of the average motor unit in a muscle determines how precisely contractions of that muscle can be altered. This limitation can be appreciated when the size of the average motor unit in the thigh muscle and the intrinsic eye muscle are compared: the former contains many thousands of fibres whilst the latter contains only three (Karpovich and Sinning 1971).

The intrafusal fibres (or muscle spindles) bear sensory receptors which fire in response to static and dynamic changes in muscle length. Activity in the *gamma efferent* pathway causes intrafusal fibres to contract, and this action is important in preserving *afferent* information from the sensory receptors. If gamma efferent activity is absent, sensory signals from the muscle spindles gradually cease as the muscle shortens. This 'unloading' of the spindle can be prevented if a compensatory shortening of the intrafusal fibres is instigated (Fig. 2). If gamma efferent activity is programmed so that the spindle is always kept at the length at which it is maximally sensitive to changes in the contraction of the muscle, optimally precise information about the performance will be retained.

Reflex Activity

The afferent output from a muscle spindle can trigger muscular contractions directly. These automatic reactions are important for explaining postural control in neurologically normal persons and they are of great importance for understanding the postural abnormalities and movement difficulties shown by spastic individuals. The stretch reflex will be discussed because of its importance in regulating posture and because it figures in models of movement control: the tendon jerk will be discussed because of its use as a clinical index.

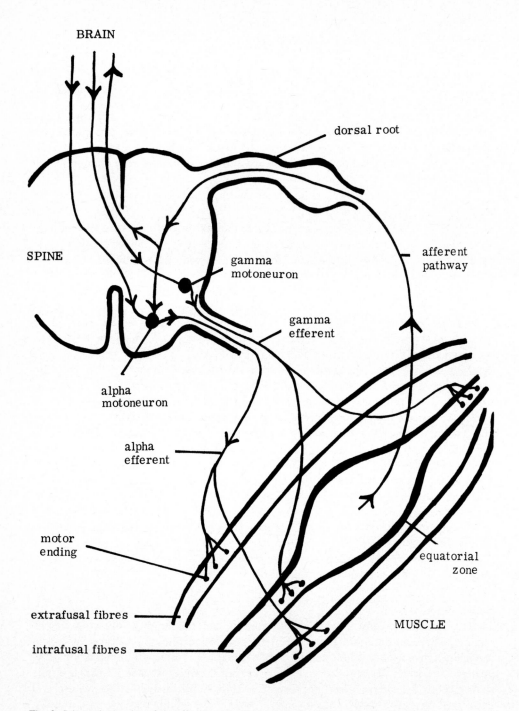

Fig. 1. Schematic drawing of the efferent and afferent pathways that supply muscle fibres.

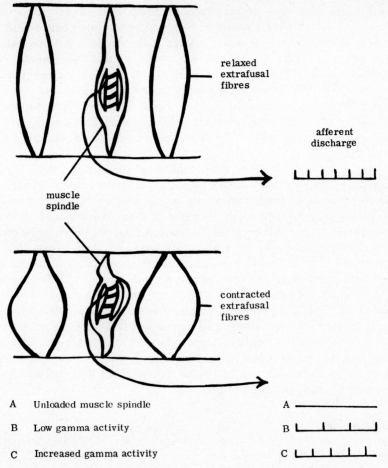

Fig. 2. The effects of muscular contraction and gamma efferent activity on the frequency of afferent discharge from the muscle spindle receptors.

The tendon jerk is elicited by a sharp tap to the muscle tendon. This stimulus lengthens the muscle and evokes rapid synchronised firing of the primary receptors in the muscle spindle. A direct spinal pathway is present and the impulses which are produced cause alpha motoneurons to fire. The muscle which was originally lengthened by the tap is observed to contract.

The stretch reflex also brings about the compensatory contraction of a muscle, but in this instance the stimulus is slow, passive stretching of the muscle. The afferent firing which results activates alpha motoneurons supplying the muscle which was stretched and inhibits activity in the antagonist muscle. When body position is altered, the force that is acting on a skeletal muscle may change. The stretch reflex provides a mechanism for compensating for any resultant changes in muscle length.

Recent evidence (Marsden *et al.* 1973) strongly suggests that the stretch reflex in man is mediated by a transcortical loop and not a spinal pathway. Phillips (1969) investigated neuromuscular control in baboons, and postulated that the spinal stretch reflex 'has been overlaid in the course of evolution by a transcortical circuit'. Evarts (1973) believes that he has seen a transcortical loop functioning in unanaesthetised monkeys when they perform learned movements. These observations call into question the traditional view that the tendon jerk provides an adequate test of whether the stretch reflex is functioning in the human system. However, this view may be correct for some mammalian species. These interpretations do provide an explanation for why measuring resistance to passive stretch and testing the tendon jerk have sometimes provided conflicting clinical evidence for the integrity of the stretch reflex.

Long ago, Hughlings Jackson (1888) pointed out that many of the reflexes which are observed in the young infant cannot be elicited in the neurologically normal adult but may reappear in the senile patient. He concluded that the higher centres in the nervous system suppress activity in the lower centres. Wiesendanger *et al.* (1974) suggest that superimposed cortical circuits inhibit some transcortical reflexes. This inhibition may be destroyed by pathological changes, and, when this occurs, particular kinds of reflex activity reappear. Individuals who have suffered a lesion in the precentral motor area may show forms of tactile grasping. When an object is placed in his hand, the patient grasps it reflexively and he must make a considerable effort before he is able to counter this. Whatever useful functions reflexes serve for the developing child, it is clear that they also impose restrictions on the responses which can be made to certain situations. Once reflex activity has been inhibited, the individual is able to achieve a greater flexibility of response. For example, once tactile grasping has been checked, the individual can learn to keep his hand flat and examine objects which are placed on it.

Sensory Information

Various sources of information are available for evaluating neuromuscular activity (Connolly 1969). *Reafferent* information is the term used to distinguish those afferent signals which are initiated by voluntary muscular activity. Reafferent signals are produced by sensory receptors in the muscle spindles, tendons, joints and skin. The nature and precision of the information produced by different receptors varies (Mountcastle 1968). In contrast, *exafferent* information is triggered by external stimuli. When a muscle is passively stretched, receptors in the muscle spindles produce exafferent information. The visual monitoring of a movement also provides exafferent information about the performance. Central signals are available which reflect the efferent programme which is creating the movement. This source of information has been labelled the 'efference copy' (von Holst and Mittelstaedt 1950) or 'corollary discharge' (Sperry 1950). An appropriate selection from amongst the sources of information that are available can lead to improved monitoring and better error detection. Paillard and Brouchon (1974) demonstrated that proprioceptive information contributed to the accurate location of a moving limb, whilst visual information was best for evaluating a stable position.

Held and Bauer (1974) have emphasised the vital rôle played by visual information in calibrating movement signals so that they become useful for judging the progress of a movement. Monkeys that are not allowed to see their limbs moving are prevented from calibrating the efference copy, exafferent cues or reafferent signals in terms of the movements actually achieved. In consequence, they are unable to reach accurately with their arms. These authors point out that normal body growth (including that of effector organs and receptors) must act as a chronic form of rearrangement which will necessitate that movement signals are recalibrated regularly.

The wealth of information sources which are available provides the possibility that when some are abnormal or damaged, the individual will learn to concentrate on others and so gain better control. Held and Bauer (1974) showed that monkeys which had been prevented from seeing their limbs could be taught to make specific arm reaches using an operant conditioning technique. That the monkeys showed poor generalisation when the object to be reached for was moved was attributed to the fact that the available movement signals had never been calibrated. It is important to note that the monkeys were able to learn to produce the chosen movements with accuracy and reliability.

Bossom (1974) provides an excellent review of studies designed to investigate what level of movement control is possible when afferent information from a limb is blocked. He concludes that the recovery shown by monkeys after complete dorsal rhizotomy depends upon the post-operative care that they receive and on how much encouragement is given to the monkeys to attempt movements. Immediately after the operation these animals spend much of their time looking at their limbs. Using visual information, they are able to learn to locomote and to reach for objects. They have difficulty in grasping objects effectively: one reason for this is that they do not use their thumbs (see Fig. 3). At this stage they are able to bring their hand to their mouth directly, but, in general, the movements they display lack normal co-ordination and have been described as 'ataxic' and 'clumsy'. However, with careful training they can achieve more normal control. Monkeys have been trained to pick up raisins using the thumb and fore-finger in opposition. There is also evidence that these animals can use 'efference copy' information, *i.e.* they are able to reach accurately for objects when visual monitoring is prevented. Bossom (1974) points to a number of difficulties in interpreting such studies, one of which is that dorsal rhizotomy may not eliminate proprioceptive information completely. His studies strongly suggest, however, that some movement control can be achieved when only efference copy and visual information sources are available.

Motor Control

Connolly (see Chapter 8) outlines the difficulties of attempting to characterise actions in terms of muscular contractions and of assuming that people plan actions in terms of the movements which are used to achieve them. Teuber (1974) provides an example which illustrates these points. When individuals who had suffered upper-arm amputation were asked to contract either the biceps or the triceps muscle they were able to do so without difficulty and Sherringtonian inhibition of the antagonist was observed. However, when asked to contract these muscles simultaneously they were unable to do so. When the instruction was changed and they were asked to make a 'phantom fist', good co-activation of these muscles was observed. The patient knew

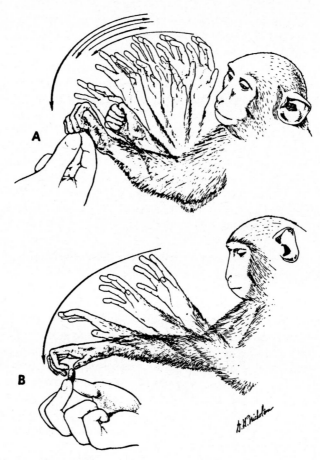

Fig. 3. A: shows shovel grasp in monkeys following motor recovery after brachial dorsal rhizotomy. The oscillation of the arm toward and away from food is seen only in some animals. B: shows dexterity seen in a normal arm extension and grasp using finger and thumb opposition.

how to make a fist, but this knowledge was not coded in terms of the muscular contractions which were used to achieve the action. From the viewpoint of the performer this is eminently sensible, for he moves muscles in order to achieve actions, and improvement for him is equated with a visibly refined performance. He has no reason to be aware of muscle activity unless this is a specific requirement of the task (Hefferline 1958, Basmajian 1963). When relevant augmented feedback is provided, the subject is capable of learning to code and regulate muscular activity *per se.*

Even though the individual is unlikely to be aware of his performance in these terms, it is clear that a movement will be improved if he is able to achieve faster, more precise muscular contractions. One factor which determines how well an action is executed by a limb which has not been used for this purpose before is how accurately the subject is able to regulate muscular contractions within it. If the individual is unable to control the position of his foot, he will be unable to write with it even though he can write accurately with his hand. Therefore there is good reason to try to distinguish between good and poor strategies for regulating muscular activity and good and poor methods of dealing with errors which occur. This is particularly true in the case of spastic individuals, for they are likely to have difficulty in achieving accurate contractions.

The control exhibited in executing a muscular contraction may be judged in terms of whether the correct pattern of force is achieved and in terms of whether accuracy is safeguarded by making some provision for detecting errors and correcting them. A number of models have been offered to explain how well-executed contractions are achieved. Merton (1953) believed that alpha efferent activity was employed only when urgent movements were called for. In his model, good control depended on programming gamma efferent activity appropriately. He believed that when the appropriate misalignment between intrafusal and extrafusal fibres was achieved, afferent output from the muscle spindle receptors would trigger the degree of contraction which was desired. In this system, changes in external force were compensated for quickly and accurately by reflexive lengthening or shortening of the muscle. Information which was not available at this time indicates that the afferent output from a spindle may stimulate activity in a number of muscles. It is therefore difficult to see how this mechanism could be used to programme precise movements (Lundberg 1959). Neither has it been established that there is sufficient gain across this pathway for muscular activity to be initiated by gamma efferent activity alone (Matthews 1966, 1967; Granit 1968).

The model outlined by Phillips (1969) proposed that motor control depends upon the appropriate *coactivation* of alpha and gamma efferent activity. This model owes a great deal to the ideas of Matthews (1964) and Granit (1955, 1968). In this system, alpha efferent activity is programmed to achieve the degree of contraction which is desired and gamma efferent activity plays a vital rôle in error detection and error correction. Two systems of error correction are included. The first is a system of reflexive compensation similar to that proposed by Merton (1953). When gamma efferent activity has been used to adjust the sensitivity of the muscle spindle to the appropriate level, any change in external force will trigger the amount of alpha motoneuron activity which is required to compensate for its effect. When studying respiratory action, Corda *et al.* (1965) showed that alpha and gamma neurons of the intercostal muscles are indeed coactivated. Respiratory obstruction was observed to produce increases in spindle discharge which resulted in the compensatory increase in alpha motoneuron activity. The work of Vallbo (1971) offers support for Phillips' model and also challenges models which include gamma efferent initiation of contractions. He made direct recordings of spindle afferent activity in hand muscles and showed that spindle acceleration occurs after the onset of electromyographic activity.

The second system of error correction proposed by Phillips requires a central representation of afferent output from the muscle receptors. Careful programming of gamma efferent activity is required to avoid spindle 'unloading' and so preserve precise afferent information. In the case of skilled movements, Phillips suggests that 'signals of mismatch', indicating deviations from the movement which was planned,

41

will trigger the required adjustments to efferent activity directly. Evarts (1967) isolated a large pyramidal cell whose firing reflected flexor muscle force, not flexor muscle displacement. Commenting on this finding, Phillips (1969) stated:

"One may hazard the speculation that the increased discharge of the pyramidal tract cell ... was in response to a signal of mismatch between intended and actual displacement. Whether this signal is a crude one from the muscle spindles or whether the mismatch has been computed by the cerebellum is still unknown; nor, in this experiment can the contribution of joints, skin and vision be assessed. But however 'instructed' the corticomotoneuronal projection would transfer the 'instruction' for increased force to the alpha motoneurons with maximum directness."

Further studies (Phillips *et al.*, 1971) suggest that these changes in pyramidal tract cell firing are not brought about by crude 'signals of mismatch' produced by muscle receptors.

In Phillips' model, alpha efferent activity is programmed to achieve the desired movements, and systems of error correction are used to ensure that this movement is realised. The term 'servo-assisted' has been used to describe such a system. Better movement control will follow if the person isolates a more accurate and economic programme of alpha efferent activity and if he learns to exploit the systems of error correction which are available to him so that mistakes are detected quickly and remedied accurately.

A further complexity to this system has been uncovered by Merton (1974), who studied the servo action which occurs when voluntary flexion of the top joint of the thumb is obstructed unexpectedly. He used local anaesthetic to block tactile afferent information from the thumb: this procedure does not interfere with activity in the muscle spindles of the flexor pollicis longus because this muscle is situated in the fore-arm. When tactile information was blocked by anaesthetic, servo action was reduced and sometimes abolished. Merton suggests a system of 'tactile gating' to explain these results. Afferent impulses from the muscle spindles return to the cortex but they do not necessarily gain access to cortical neurons to stimulate them and so complete the servo-loop. The degree of access is variable and determines the degree of servo-action which is observed. Access is facilitated by (or may even depend on) tactile impulses from the part which is moved. Merton believes that 'tactile gating' may serve the function of focussing servo action in fine movements, a need which was recognised by Phillips (1969).

Newsom and Sears (1970) studied the intercostal stretch reflex. They showed that the initial response to increased load was not excitation, as predicted by servo theory, but rather brief inhibition was observed before the compensatory activity began. They speculated that compensation is delayed so that the significance of an unexpected event can be analysed centrally and a choice of response made. Hammond (1960) showed that subjects were able to regulate the stretch reflex so as to comply with instructions which they had been given. If asked to resist a load, the stretch reflex was enhanced. If asked to 'let go', the stretch reflex was inhibited. These studies suggest that when the individual has sufficient time, or prior knowledge, he is able to modify reflex activity so that it contributes to the action in progress. This type of economy was found by Evarts (1973) to characterise the performances of a highly trained monkey. The task for the monkey was to pull or push a handle, as instructed at the beginning of a trial. The signal to begin the movement consisted of a displacement of the handle, either towards or away from the subject. On some trials, the displacement of the handle provoked tendon jerk and stretch reflex activity in accord with the movement signified. The volume of reflex activity observed in these situations was markedly greater than during trials in which any reflex activity would have been counter-productive. Changes in motor cortex neuron firing were observed when the instruction was given and before the handle was displaced. These changes altered the bias on the spinal reflex mechanism and modulated the transcortical servo-loop: reflex activity was enhanced when conducive to the required movement and suppressed when it functioned against the action planned. The skilled performer had preprogrammed his system so as to minimise the effects of unwanted changes, and, at the same time, to capitalise on any helpful changes that occurred.

Programming Movements

Megaw (1974) outlines one method for investigating the motor programme which underlies a movement. It is based on the assumption that the programme reflects a hierarchy of decisions which have been made about the movement, decisions such as which muscles are to be active and how long each contraction should last. If a hierarchy is accepted, then it follows that a lower level in the programme will be changed more easily than a higher level. Megaw studied how the time taken to modify an action (refractory period) varies with the type of modification which is demanded, and used these data to achieve a *post hoc* definition of the motor programme. He concluded that the actual muscles involved in a movement are programmed at a high level. At a lower level, the broad sequence of muscle activity is specified. At a lower level still, more precise temporal features are programmed, such as the interval between activity in one muscle group and the next. At the lowest level, the duration and strength of each contraction is specified. Speeding up a movement, which can be achieved by reducing the time taken to execute component contractions, is therefore achieved more easily than slowing down the same movement because this requires that the sequence of activity is altered so that the antagonist can be introduced to slow the movement.

In the short term, what is important is whether the subject can compose a movement programme which is adequate for the task he is facing. In the long term, what may be important is whether he has learned anything which he can generalise to new tasks. As a result, one would expect to see the individual developing consistent ways of analysing problems, consistent ways of monitoring actions and evaluating them, and sterotyped patterns of movement. The term 'subroutine' has been used to describe part of an action programme which reappears in a variety of such programmes (Bruner 1970, Connolly 1970). Kots and Syrovegin (1966) demonstrated that subjects used consistent patterns of joint movement to execute arm flexions and extensions. They compared the rate of change in angle at the elbow with that at the wrist and found that any individual produced only five to seven ratios. There was a wide variation in the particular ratios shown by the different subjects studied, but the number used by any individual was small. The limited range of responses is not caused

43

by any mechanical coupling in the system, rather it indicates that the subject has isolated a small number of responses which are useful in a variety of situations.

Attempts have been made to define and isolate units of movement. If a suitable system is achieved, it may prove useful for distinguishing between good and poor solutions to a motor problem. This type of analysis may also provide information on the changes which occur as motor control is developed. One system of definition is based on the fact that movements consist of a series of ballistic elements. Each element is pre-programmed and can be revised only after it has been completed and its performance has been evaluated. A movement unit can therefore be defined operationally in terms of the fact that it cannot be modified during its execution. Brooks (1974) studied two types of movement which differ in their acceleration profile. In the majority of cases he found that 'continuous movements' were not affected when movement cues were manipulated during their performance, whereas 'discontinuous movements' were revised while they were being performed if new information was received. Moreover, he found that discontinuous movements are made up of steps that resemble small continuous movements. Obvious advantages would be gained if movement units could be distinguished in terms of their acceleration characteristics, and research is needed to study whether the duration of continuous movements increases as an action is performed more skilfully. Encouragement is provided by Brooks' observation that 'Monkeys tended to use discontinuous movements when the task situation had been changed or when they were unsure what was expected of them for any other reason'.

A number of advantages are likely to follow if a movement is completed using fewer units. As the person is spending less time setting up the transition from one unit to the next, the movement is likely to be faster and will possibly require less cognitive effort. Support for this comes from the work of Leonard (1959) and Welford (1974) in which they forced subjects to string responses together whilst preventing the subject from spending time in monitoring whether responses had been completed successfully. The responses chosen were over-learned movements which the subject was able to pre-programme accurately. Instead of the stimulus for the next response being given after the completion of the last one, it was introduced before, or at the instant when, the previous response was begun. This schedule evoked an uncanny feeling in the subjects of being automated. Subjects reported that they felt unhurried and that they felt as though they were not having to consciously order their actions. Their performance on the task was smoother than that observed on a normal schedule, presumably because the performance was not being interrupted to check that responses had been completed successfully. In terms of the definition offered above, the subject is being forced into adopting larger units of movement. This is presumably an engineered example of what happens normally when better movement control is achieved. The subject learns to pre-programme larger packages of efferent activity accurately and so the movement becomes smoother and faster. The model proposed by Phillips (1969) fits in well with this analysis. His systems for error correction mean that some errors will be dealt with automatically while the unit is in progress; deviations which are not handled in this way will be corrected quickly when the pre-programmed activity is finished. The initiation of the next unit is therefore delayed only minimally.

A basic feature of the spastic syndrome is hyperactivity of the spinal motoneurons (Dimitrijevič and Nathan 1967). Landau and Clare (1964) used the H reflex to measure directly the threshold for activity of alpha motoneurons. In hemiplegic patients, they found that those which supplied impaired muscles had abnormally low thresholds. One explanation which has been put forward to account for the heightened sensitivity of the motoneurons is that the gamma efferents which supply spastic muscles are hyperactive. Walshe (1924) demonstrated that spasticity can be abolished by intramuscular injections of procaine. Confirmatory results were obtained by Rushworth (1960) who treated patients whose spasticity was not accompanied by flexor spasms. He injected procaine either into the muscles or around a major nerve and found that this had the effect of abolishing the hyperactive stretch reflex for a short time. During this period, voluntary power remained unaffected. In some patients, this effect could not be achieved and it was assumed that alpha rigidity was present. Rushworth concluded that procaine produces this effect because it blocks activity in the thinner gamma efferent fibres whilst not interfering with activity in the thicker alpha efferents. Certain objections have been raised against this interpretation. Landau et al. (1960) studied the action of procaine, but could find no evidence which suggested that spasticity is caused by excessive gamma efferent activity. Meltzer et al. (1963) studied stretch reflex activity in spastic monkeys and concluded that gamma efferent activity did not provide a sufficient explanation for the hyperreflexia that was present. Walshe (1924) originally ascribed the action of procaine in abolishing spasticity to the fact that it blocks the afferent output from a muscle, and Gassel and Diamantopoulos (1964) revived this explanation to account for their own results.

If spasticity is caused by excessive gamma efferent activity, some alleviation would be expected when posterior spinal roots are cut, for it is these fibres which transmit impulses from the muscle spindles to the alpha motoneurons. Working with human patients, Foerster (1911) found that dorsal rhizotomy did depress spasticity, and in some cases abolished it. Subsequent investigations have shown that the condition recurs in a large number of cases (Lehmann 1936, Freeman and Heimburger 1948). However, the possibility that the surgery may create fresh problems of imbalance and loss of inhibition makes it difficult to interpret these findings.

Mild spasticity is demonstrated only when the muscle is stretched rapidly. This suggests that the dynamic spindle receptors are hypersensitive in this condition (Jansen 1962). Two types of gamma efferent have been identified. The thicker dynamic gamma efferents bias the output of dynamic spindle receptors; the static gamma efferents alter the responsiveness of static spindle receptors. The characteristics of mild spasticity are consistent with it being caused by hyperactivity in dynamic gamma efferents. In severe cases of spasticity the tonic reflexes are sometimes so strong that dynamic reflexes are not exhibited. When treating such patients, Rushworth (1960) found that tendon jerks could be elicited after an appropriate level of procaine block had been administered. Rushworth believed that this effect was achieved because the procaine was blocking activity only in the thinner (static) gamma efferents. Whether this is correct, or whether the procaine is actually blocking afferent output from the static receptors, cannot be judged. In summary, the spastic syndrome is known to involve hyperactive alpha motoneurons. Although many observations support the view that gamma efferent hyperactivity is also involved, others caution against this opinion.

Hyperreflexia

A number of important consequences stem from the fact that the alpha motoneurons which supply spastic muscles have a lowered threshold for activity. The contractions which are recorded in spastic muscles may be abnormally strong, and contractions can be elicited by stimuli which are normally innocuous. The postures observed in spastic persons are sometimes highly abnormal: this is due in part to the fact that spastic muscles exhibit a hyperactive stretch reflex. The pull of gravity is therefore sufficient to cause a marked contraction in the muscles which oppose it (the anatomical flexors). The continuous activity which is present in these muscles may limit severely the movements which the person is able to achieve. Antagonist muscles may be unable to overcome this tonus and so they appear weak and, indeed, may become weak. The conditions therefore exist for limb deformities to develop. When a spastic limb is passively moved, strong opposition is felt. Tasks such as dressing are therefore difficult to achieve. If stretching of the muscle is continued, it may yield suddenly and movement will become possible; this is known as the 'clasp-knife' phenomenon. Golgi receptors in the tendon respond to changes of tension in the muscle attached to it. The afferent output which is produced by these receptors serves to inhibit contraction of the active muscle and to facilitate activity in its antagonist. The clasp-knife phenomenon is assumed to occur when the force in the antagonist becomes greater than that in the muscle which is being stretched. The two forms of reflex activity which are described above work in opposition; this serves to limit the range of movements which can be achieved. The extreme case is observed when the spastic limb is held in a rigid position because of the presence of continuously counteracted and counteracting contractions.

Bobath (1966) drew a distinction between *abnormal* and *primitive* reflexes in the spastic syndrome. Primitive reflexes are defined as those which are observed in neurologically normal infants. Abnormal reflexes, on the other hand, are never observed in the normal neuromusculature. The Moro reflex is seen when young babies are startled: it is characterised by wide abduction of the arms, extension at the elbows and wrists and abduction and extension of the fingers and thumbs. This reflex is retained by some spastic individuals and makes it difficult for them to maintain equilibrium in a sitting position.

In the experimental studies which are reported later (Chapters 6 and 7), the ability of spastic subjects to regulate movements of the wrist was assessed while the subjects were seated. It is likely that a number of difficulties were created for them by hyperreflexia of the spastic muscles and the presence of abnormal and primitive reflexes. The force of gravity may produce prominent flexion of the wrist joint. If asked to extend his wrist from this posture, the spastic subject is likely to experience difficulty for reasons which have been outlined already. If only a slight flexion of the wrist is required, the subject will first have to inhibit some of the resting tonus in the flexor muscle. Voluntary movement of any kind is likely to be impeded (and possibly prevented) by contractions produced by the stretch and clasp-knife reflexes. Many potential sources of interference are present in the spastic neuromuscular system, which must be controlled if movements are to be safeguarded. For example, wrist movements can be triggered by activity in the ipsilateral or contralateral limb. Movements of the head can also interfere with the planned wrist movement. The asymmetrical tonic neck reflex is triggered when the head is turned to one side, and results in extension of the limbs on the side to which the head is turned and flexion of the opposite limbs. In summary, the task facing the spastic individual is not simply one of trying to understand the instructions and of isolating a movement which is appropriate. He must also try to maintain a controlled posture (which he often finds difficult) and he must try to avoid or check patterns of interference and patterns of excess activity.

Motor Control

In the models of skilled movement which have been discussed, afferent feedback plays a vital rôle. The information produced from the muscle spindles may be used to evaluate a contraction and if gamma efferent activity has been used to bias this output appropriately, the afferent signals will produce corrections directly. If gamma efferent or spindle afferent activity is abnormal in the spastic system, this is likely to impede good motor control. Harrison and Connolly (1971) pointed to the fact that spindle afferent signals may be difficult to decipher and so the spastic person may be unable to use these to judge whether contractions have been achieved successfully. Indeed these individuals may never have had the opportunity to associate afferent signals with the muscles which produce them. The welter of contractions which can follow when the spastic person produces a movement will make it difficult for him to learn to ascribe particular signals to specific muscles correctly. Without this understanding, he will be unable to use these signals to identify sources of interference and so achieve a functional definition of his complex neuromusculature. The spastic individual is therefore likely to experience difficulty in learning to produce accurate motor programmes, detect movement errors, and control sources of interference. In short, he will probably not realise his full potential for movement control under everyday conditions. Electromyographic information indicates which muscles are active and the contractile strength present in particular muscles. In later studies (Chapter 7), this was used to provide spastic individuals with augmented feedback to help them code inherent movement signals, and under such conditions they acquired better motor control.

Alpha motoneuron hyperactivity will limit the types of movement which can be achieved. Hyperreflexia is one effect which has already been discussed. Alpha motoneuron hyperactivity will also prevent the subject from controlling fine levels of contraction. Harrison and Connolly (1971) and Harrison (1973) showed that spastic subjects were able to reduce excess neuromuscular activity when electromyographic feedback was provided. This index allowed the spastic subjects to isolate the muscle which was to be controlled and to receive unambiguous information about whether attempts to suppress hyperactivity were successful. The opportunity to evaluate accurately an attempt to improve motor control may have been totally novel for the spastic person. The possibility therefore exists that spastic individuals have the capability of achieving good motor control if the appropriate form of training can be found.

SUMMARY

The picture that emerges is one in which the spastic individual is faced with the problem of having to learn to use a functionally complex neuromusculature when his ability to programme activity may be limited and his ability to monitor activity impaired. Even if he is incapable of damping alpha motoneuron hyperactivity, some improvement in control should be possible. It seems likely, however, that he may need special training to help him isolate optimal efferent programmes and strategies for minimising reflexive interference. Studies of normal motor control have shown that central control of reflex activity can be achieved. It therefore seems a reasonable hope that spastic persons are capable of suppresing hyperactivity and hyperreflexia if only suitable training schedules can be found.

Acknowledgements

Fig. 3 is taken from 'Movement without Proprioception' by J. Bossom (Brain Research, 71, 299) and is reproduced by kind permission of Elsevier Scientific Publishers.

REFERENCES

Basmajian, J. V. (1963) 'Control and training of individual motor units.' *Science,* **141,** 440.

Bobath, K. (1966) *Motor Deficit in Patients with Cerebral Palsy.* Clinics in Developmental Medicine, no. 23. London: Spastics International Medical Publications with Heinemann Medical.

Bossom , J, (1974) 'Movement without proprioception.' *Brain Research,* **71,** 285.

Brooks, V. B. (1974) 'Some examples of programmed limb movements.' *Brain Research,* **71,** 299.

Bruner, J. (1970) 'The growth and structure of skill.' *In* Connolly, K. (Ed.) *Mechanisms of Motor Skill Development.* C.A.S.D.S. Study Group on the Mechanisms of Motor Skill Development. London and New York: Academic Press.

Connolly, K. (1969) 'Sensory-motor coordination: Mechanisms and plans.' *In* Wolff, P. H., Mac Keith, R. (Eds.) *Planning for Better Learning.* Clinics in Developmental Medicine, no. 33. London: Spastics International Medical Publications with Heinemann Medical.

—— (1970) 'Skill development: problems and plans.' *In* Connolly, K. (Ed.) *Mechanisms of Motor Skill Development.* C.A.S.D.S. Study Group on Mechanisms of Motor Skill Development. London and New York: Academic Press.

Corda, M., Eklund, G., Euler, C. von (1965) 'External intercostal and phrenic alpha-motor responses to changes in respiratory load.' *Acta Physiologica Scandinavica,* **63,** 391.

Dimitrijević, M. R., Nathan, P. W. (1967) 'Studies of spasticity in man. I. Some features of spasticity.' *Brain,* **90,** 1.

Evarts, E. V. (1967) 'Representation of movements and muscles by pyramidal tract neurons of the precentral motor cortex.' *In* Yahr, M. D., Purpura, D. P. (Eds.) *Neurophysiological Basis of Normal and Abnormal Motor Activities.'* Hewlett, N. Y.: Raven Press.

—— (1973) 'Motor cortex reflexes associated with learned movement.' *Science,* **179,** 501.

Foerster, O. (1911) 'Die behandlung spasticher Lähmungen durch Resektion hinterer Rüchenmarks-wurzeln.' *Ergebnisse der Chirurgie und Orthopädei*, **2**, 174.

Freeman, L. W., Heimburger, R. F. (1948) 'The surgical relief of spasticity in paraplegic patients. II. Peripheral nerve section, posterior rhizotomy, and other procedures.' *Journal of Neurosurgery*, **5**, 556.

Gassel, M. M., Diamantopoulos, E. (1964) 'The effect of procaine nerve block on neuromuscular reflex regulation in man. An appraisal of the role of the fusimotor system.' *Brain*, **87**, 729

Granit, R. (1955) *Receptors and Sensory Perception.* Newhaven: Yale University Press.

—— (1968) 'The functional role of the muscle spindle's primary end organs.' *Proceedings of the Royal Society of Medicine*, **61**, 69.

Hammond, P. H. (1960) 'An experimental study of servo action in human muscular control.' *In Proceedings of the Third International Conference on Medical Electronics*, London: Iliffe; Springfield, Ill.: C. C. Thomas, p. 190.

Harrison, A. (1973) 'Studies of neuromuscular control in spastic persons.' Unpublished Ph.D. thesis, Sheffield University.

—— Connolly, K. (1971) 'The conscious control of fine levels of neuromuscular firing in spastic and normal subjects.' *Developmental Medicine and Child Neurology*, **13**, 762.

Hefferline, R. F. (1958) 'The role of proprioception in the control of behavior.' *Transactions of the New York Academy of Sciences*, **141**, 440.

Held, R., Bauer, J. A. (1974) 'Development of sensorially-guided reaching in infant monkeys.' *Brain Research*, **71**, 265.

Jackson, J. H. (1888) Discussion at the Neurological Society on muscular hypertonicity in paralysis, on July 7th, 1888. *Brain*, **10**, 312.

Jansen, J. K. S. (1962) 'Spasticity—functional aspects.' *Acta Neurologica Scandinavica*, **38** (Suppl. 3) 41.

Karpovich, P. V., Sinning, W. E. (1971) *Physiology of Muscular Activity*, 7th ed. Philadelphia: Saunders.

Kots, Ya. M., Syrovegin, A. V. (1966) 'Fixed set of variants of the interaction of muscles of two joints used in the execution of simple voluntary movements.' *(Russian) Biofizika*, **11**, 1061.

Landau, W. M., Weaver, R. A., Hornbein, T. F. (1960) 'Fusimotor nerve function in man. Differential nerve block studies in normal subjects and in spasticity and rigidity.' *Archives of Neurology*, **3**, 10.

Landau, W. M., Clare, M. H. (1964) 'Fusimotor function. Part VI. H reflex, tendon jerk and reinforcement in hemiplegia.' *Archives of Neurology*, **10**, 128.

Lehmann, W. (1936) 'Chirurgische Therapie bei Erkrankungen und Verletzungen des Nervensystems.' *In* Bumke, O., Foerster, O. (Eds.) *Handbuch der Neurologie*, Berlin: Springer.

Leonard, J. A. (1959) 'Tactual choice reations.' *Quarterly Journal of Experimental Psychology*, **11**, 76.

Lundberg, A. (1959) 'Integrative significance of patterns of connections made by muscle afferents in the spinal cord.' *XXI International Congress of Physiological Sciences, Buenos Aires*, p. 100.

Marsden, C. D., Merton, P. A., Morton, H. B. (1973) 'Is the human stretch reflex spinal rather than cortical?' *Lancet*, **i**, 759.

Matthews, P. B. C. (1964) 'Muscle spindles and their motor control.' *Physiological Review*, **44**, 219.

—— (1966) 'The reflex excitation of the soleus muscle of the decerebrate cat caused by vibration applied to its tendon.' *Journal of Physiology*, **184**, 450.

—— (1967) 'The reflex response to muscle vibration in the decerebrate cat.' *Journal of Physiology*, **192**, 18.

Megaw, E. D. (1974) 'Possible modification to a rapid on-going programmed manual response.' *Brain Research*, **71**, 425.

Meltzer, G. E., Hunt, R. S., Landau, W. M. (1963) 'Fusimotor function. Part III. The spastic monkey.' *Archives of Neurology*, **9**, 133.

Merton, P. A. (1953) *Speculation on the Servo-Control of Movement.* London: Churchill.

—— (1974) 'The properties of the human muscle servo.' *Brain Research*, **71**, 475.

Mountcastle, V. B. (1968) 'Physiology of sensory receptors: introduction to sensory processes.' *In* Mountcastle, V. B. (Ed.) *Medical Physiology.* St. Louis: Mosby.

Newsom Davis, J., Sears, T. A. (1970) 'The proprioceptive reflex control of the intercostal muscles during their voluntary activation.' *Journal of Physiology*, **209**, 711.

Paillard, J., Brouchon, M. (1974) 'A proprioceptive contribution to the spatial encoding of position cues for ballistic movements.' *Brain Research*, **71**, 273.

Phillips, C. G. (1969) 'Motor apparatus of the baboon's hand.' *Proceedings of the Royal Society, Series B.*, **173**, 141.

—— Powell, T. P. S., Wiesdanger, M. (1971) 'Projection from low threshold muscle afferents of hand and forearm to area 3a of baboon's cortex.' *Journal of Physiology*, **217**, 419.

Rushworth, G. (1960) 'Spasticity and rigidity: an experimental study and review.' *Journal of Neurology, Neurosurgery and Psychiatry*, **23**, 99.

Sharrard, W. J. W. (1974) 'Observations on paralysis, muscle growth and bone deformity.' *In* Zorab, P. A. (Ed.) *Scoliosis and Muscle. Proceedings of a Fourth Symposium held at the Cardiothoracic Institute, Brompton Hospital, London, 1973.* Research Monograph no. 4. London: Spastics International Medical Publications with Heinemann Medical.

Sperry, R. W. (1950) 'Neural basis of the spontaneous optokinetic response produced by visual inversion.' *Journal of Comparative and Physiological Psychology,* **43,** 482.

Teuber, H. L. (1974) 'Key problems in the programming of movements. Panel discussion.' *Brain Research,* **71,** 567.

Vallbo, A. B. (1971) 'Muscle spindle response at the onset of isometric voluntary contractions in man. Time differences between fusimotor and skeletomotor effects.' *Journal of Physiology,* **218,** 405.

von Holst, E., Mittlestaedt, H. (1950) 'Das Reafferenzprinzip.' *Naturwissenschaften,* **37,** 464.

Walshe, F. M. R. (1924) 'Observations on the nature of muscular rigidity of paralysis agitans and on its relationship to tremor.' *Brain,* **47,** 159.

Welford, A. T. (1974) 'On the sequencing of action.' *Brain Research,* **71,** 381.

Wiesendanger, M., Seguin, J. J., Kunzle, H. (1974) 'The supplementary motor area—a control system for posture?' *In* Stein, R. B. (Ed.) *Control of Posture and Locomotion.* New York: Plenum.

CHAPTER SIX

Studies of Neuromuscular Control
in Normal and Spastic Individuals

ANN HARRISON

In the studies which follow, electromyography was used to provide a measure of muscular activity. When a muscle contracts, ionic changes take place which reflect the strength of the contraction (Lenman and Ritchie 1970). Electromyography records these potential changes and can therefore be used to assess which muscles are active during a movement; it can also be used to log increases and decreases in the activity of a specific muscle.

Two major forms of electrode are available for detecting electromyographic (EMG) activity. Needle electrodes inserted into a muscle can be used to detect very small changes in contractile strength. This system must be used if motor unit firings are to be recorded. The fact that a needle electrode records from only a small area of the muscle means that the activity which it transmits may not be representative of that occurring in the muscle as a whole. A more appropriate means for assessing over-all activity in a muscle is to use surface electrodes, which was the technique adopted in the present studies. The electrodes are attached to the skin over the muscle which is being investigated. The intervening tissues and tissue fluids are good conducting media and so EMG changes can be detected at the skin surface. Surface electromyography is not sensitive to the motor unit level of activity.

Contractile strength is boosted as more motor units become active and when already-active alpha motoneurons begin to fire more frequently (Lenman and Ritchie 1970). The trained observer can use EMG recordings to assess the level of activity in a muscle and to decide whether this is increasing or decreasing. Changes in contractile strength can be quantified by integrating EMG activity. Integration is achieved by summating all the electrical activity which is recorded during a specified time period. The integrated EMG displays the summated activity occurring in successive time periods. It allows the experimenter to identify periods of relaxation and to quantify rates of increase and decrease in neuromuscular activity.

Electromyography was chosen in preference to measuring observable movements because different patterns of muscular activity can lead to indistinguishable actions. This recording technique allows one to investigate which muscles are involved in a movement and to analyse the contribution of each muscle at different stages in the action. Electromyography makes it possible to analyse why voluntary attempts at a movement are not successful and to investigate what sources of interference are disrupting the performance. EMG information may therefore help the spastic individual to achieve better movement control.

General Procedure

Silver/silver chloride surface electrodes were used. The skin was prepared by rubbing it with alcohol (to remove grease) and electrode jelly (to promote good conduction). The electrode basin was filled with electrode jelly and it was attached to the skin using adhesive plaster. The electrode placements which were used are those recommended by Davis (1952), quoted by Lippold (1967). The EMG signals were fed into a Devices AC8 preamplifier which was set to integrate the activity with a time-constant of two seconds. The integrated signal was amplified further by a Devices M4 polygraph. A permanent record was made on heat-sensitive paper, which was divided into mm divisions both horizontally and vertically. The recording paper had a useable width of 55mms. A recording speed of 5mm per sec was used.

Investigations of the motor control shown by neurologically normal and spastic individuals

A number of the difficulties which spastic persons have in controlling movements stem from the fact that a large number of muscle groups are active. It is not clear whether spastic individuals are able to control individual contractions accurately. In previous sections it was pointed out that spastic persons may never have had the opportunity to learn to programme accurately the activity within a muscle or to évaluate the contractions that are achieved. The present study was designed to investigate any difficulties which the spastic person has in controlling activity in an isolated muscle group. A major problem was to design a task which could be completed by subjects with very poor control and which would also allow levels of neuromuscular control to be differentiated and quantified.

The paradigm chosen involved asking the subjects to repeat levels of integrated electromyographic activity. An important feature of this design is that subjects were being tested on their ability to produce levels of activity which they had achieved previously. The experimenter was therefore confident that each subject was being set a task which he could perform. The accuracy which the subjects achieves is a reflection of how well he monitors and codes the contraction when he first produces it and of how well he controls muscular activity when he is asked to repeat the contraction.

Six spastic subjects were tested with age range 18 to 29 years. The neurologically normal control group consisted of six university undergraduates with age range 18 to 25 years.

Preliminary Procedure

Surface electrodes were attached to record activity in the fore-arm flexor muscle group (flexor carpi radialis and flexor digitorum sublimis). Using integrated EMG recordings, the experimenter helped the subject to identify the fore-arm flexors and to learn to contract and relax these muscles. The experimenter stressed the importance of avoiding intrinsic movements of the hand and movements of the upper arm, head and opposite limb. Various arm positions were tried until one was found which allowed the fore-arm flexors to be relaxed fully. When it was clear that the subject could comply with instructions to increase and lower activity in the fore-arm flexor muscle group, the experiment continued.

The subject was asked to tense up the fore-arm flexors as hard as he possibly could. This was repeated until a reliable maximum level of EMG activity had been established. The sensitivity of the recorder was adjusted until this integrated voltage occupied 50mms of the recording paper (Fig. 1). The maximum integrated voltage was designated tension level 10. The subject was set the task of repeating the integrated EMG voltages which represented tension levels 1 to 9. In order to avoid confusion, it should be noted that the tension levels were defined only in terms of integrated EMG activity—no assessment of muscle tension was made. Whilst an increase in EMG activity is related to an increase in muscle tension (Lippold 1967), the tension levels as defined cannot be assumed to represent accurately equal tension intervals. The term was adopted only to help subjects, for it was felt that the term 'electromyographic activity level' would be less readily understood.

The maximum integrated EMG voltage which subjects were able to produce did differ, and therefore the tension levels differed in their absolute EMG voltage from subject to subject. However, for every subject the tension levels represented the *same* proportional points along his *idiosyncratic* range from relaxation to maximum EMG activity. Therefore when subjects were asked to produce tension level 1, this represented a low activity level for all of them. When tension level 5 was set, a mid-range level of EMG activity was being demanded. When tension level 9 was set, all subjects were having to produce an EMG activity level near their maximum. This system has advantages over one in which the tension levels are defined in terms of absolute EMG voltages. Because the amount of EMG activity which is recorded

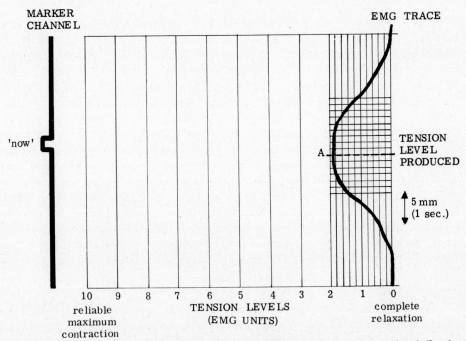

Fig. 1. Scoring technique used to assess the accuracy with which tension levels were reproduced. (Level set = 1, level produced (A) = 1.8 EMG units, error score = 0.8 EMG units, bias score = +0.8 EMG units.)

depends upon the electrode placements that are used, the system which was adopted allowed comparisons to be made across testing sessions, whereas if a set of absolute voltages had been selected, these would have had to be limited to those which the weakest subject was able to produce. In contrast, the present system allowed every subject to be tested across his full range of integrated EMG activity. Perhaps the most important criticism revolves around what it would mean to compare subjects in their ability to produce a given EMG voltage. Because subjects vary in the power that they possess, the same voltage will require different amounts of effort from them. If the example is taken of two subjects, one of whom is able to produce a maximum integrated voltage which is twice that of the other, then the weaker subject is having to make very roughly twice the effort to achieve any given voltage.

Testing Procedure

Each subject practiced the procedure in a preliminary trial which tested levels 1, 5 and 9. Five trials were then completed, each trial containing all nine tension levels in randomised order. Subjects were told not to use visual cues. At the end of each trial the subject was asked to outline the cues which he had used to judge when a tension level had been achieved.

The procedure was designed to give each subject an equivalent opportunity to code the tension level which was to be repeated. The procedure took account of the fact that some subjects were able to tense up in a controlled way and were able to hold the specified tension level without deviating, whilst other subjects consistently wavered about the target tension level.

The subject was first asked to tense up: when he reached the level which was to be repeated he was instructed to hold the tension in the muscle constant. If the subject held the target tension level accurately, he was allowed to do so for three seconds and was then told to relax. If a subject deviated from the tension level, he was told either to tense up or down as was required to regain the target level. Every time this tension level was passed through, the experimenter said 'now'. If the subject was unable to hold the tension level, he was told to relax after he had passed through the target level a total of eight times. If holding was achieved after four or less 'now' instructions, the subject was permitted to hold the target level for two seconds and was then told to relax. Only one second of holding was allowed after five, six or seven 'now' instructions had been given. As soon as relaxation was achieved, the instruction 'Repeat and tell me when' was given. The subject then tensed up until he thought that he had regained the target tension level. He was allowed to spend as much time as he wished adjusting muscular activity. When he was satisfied that he had achieved the target level, he said 'now'. The permanent record was marked at this point. The subject was then told to relax. The next level was then tested.

Results

The EMG records were used to assess the subject's attempts to reproduce the nine tension levels which had been set. A perpendicular was dropped from the record division which preceded marker activation, the EMG integrated voltage at this point was designated as the subject's response (Fig. 1). The response was measured to an accuracy of 0.2 of an EMG unit, and scores were rounded in the direction of least error. Two measures of performance were computed. The *error score* is simply the difference between the tension level which was set and that which was produced; the difference is expressed in EMG units and no account is take of whether the response was larger or smaller than the tension level which had been set. Each tension level was tested five times; the *mean error score* for a tension level indicates the average inaccuracy which was incurred during the five trials. The *bias score* was computed in exactly the same way as the error score, but this time the direction of error was noted. A positive bias score indicates that the response was greater than the target tension level. A negative bias score indicates that the subject's response was an underestimate of the tension level that had been set. The *mean bias score* reveals any tendency by the subject to consistently underestimate or overestimate the target tension level. If the underestimates for a level are as large as the overestimates, the mean bias score will be zero.

Figure 2 gives the error scores produced by the normal and spastic subject groups, and shows that the spastic subjects were less accurate than the normal subjects. The mean error for the spastic group was nearly twice as large as that recorded for the normal subjects, and greater inaccuracy was shown for all of the tension levels which were set. On analysing the variance between these data, the error scores for the two subject groups were found to be significantly different only at the ten per cent level. However, as the intra-group variance was high this might indicate a real difference in accuracy between the two subject groups. The trials were not found to differ significantly ($p > 0.05$), and no practice or fatigue effects were observed. The tension levels did not differ significantly in the accuracy with which they were reproduced ($p > 0.05$): this is probably due to the pattern of error shown by the two subject groups, for the tension levels which were reproduced most accurately by the normal subjects are just those which were performed least well by the spastic subjects. The tension level/subject group interaction was not significant ($p > 0.05$).

The bias scores recorded for the two subject groups are given in Fig. 3. The pattern which emerges is that spastic subjects have a tendency to overshoot low tension levels and to underestimate high tension levels. The normal subjects showed a tendency to overestimate the target tension levels, but this tendency was less marked when the target level was increased. An analysis of variance revealed no significant difference between the bias scores achieved by the normal and spastic subject groups ($p > 0.05$). This is not really surprising, since the spastic subjects showed both inflated negative bias and inflated positive bias and these would cancel one another out in the computation. The important factor for differentiating the performance of the two subject groups is the tension level/subject group interaction: this was found to be highly significant ($F = 11.02$; $df = 8$, [64]; $p < 0.001$)

Another way of assessing the performances achieved by spastic and normal subjects is to see how well the tension levels which were produced reflect those which were set. The group data is given in Fig. 4. It can be seen that the responses produced by the normal subjects mirrored the target levels much better than those produced by the spastic subjects. Spearman's Rank Correlation Coefficient (rs) provides a means of investigating how well the responses produced by a subject reflect the tension levels which were set. No regard is taken of the absolute errors which were made. A perfect correlation is achieved if the response given to a tension level reflects the rank order of that tension level. Fig. 5 shows the responses produced by the spastic subjects. Only four were able to achieve a significant rs score (p < 0.05), whereas all the normal subjects achieved significant rank correlations (p < 0.01).

Normal subjects reported that they had used two sorts of cue to judge when a tension level had been repeated. They used the pull produced on the wrist when the fore-arm flexors are contracted, and they also tried to estimate how much effort had been required to produce the tension level. Spastic subjects, Sp3, 4, 5 and 6 reported that they had also used effort and wrist cues to guide their performance, but Sp1 and Sp2 (the most inaccurate subjects) reported using only wrist cues.

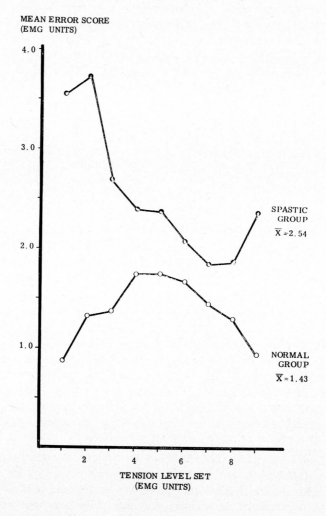

Fig. 2. The error scores shown by the neurologically normal and spastic subject groups when attempting to produce specified levels of neuromuscular activity.

56

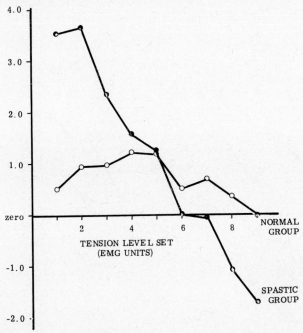

Fig. 3. The bias scores shown by the neurologically normal and spastic subject groups when attempting to produce specified levels of neuromuscular activity.

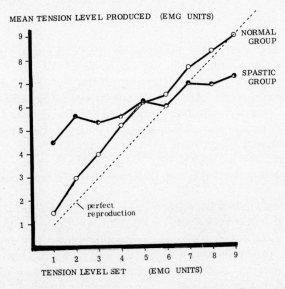

Fig. 4. The accuracy shown by neurologically normal and spastic subjects when attempting to produce specified levels of neuromuscular activity.

MEAN TENSION LEVEL PRODUCED
(EMG UNITS)

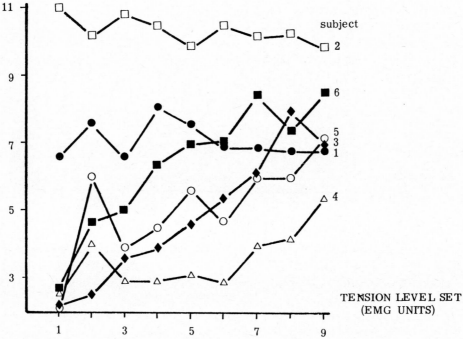

Fig. 5. The accuracy achieved by individual spastic subjects when attempting to produce specified levels of neuromuscular activity.

Discussion

In general terms, the spastic subjects were unable to match the neuromuscular control shown by the neurologically normal subjects. The spastic subjects were less accurate when repeating levels of activity in the muscle group, and two were unable to produce even a suitably ranked set of responses. None of the subjects had any difficulty in complying with the experimenter's instructions to increase or lower activity in the fore-arm flexors, which suggests that they had isolated the correct muscle group and that they had a strategy for adjusting activity within it. The question therefore remains of why the spastic subjects were unable to achieve appropriate responses when it is known that they were able to produce all the tension levels required.

The error scores indicate that the spastic subjects were most inaccurate when they were asked to repeat low tension levels. This is consistent with their having an abnormally high threshold for perceiving neuromuscular activity. In the terminology of signal detection theory, gamma hyperactivity and the contraction of other muscle groups may be producing a high level of 'noise' against which fore-arm flexor activity has to be detected. If this is so, low levels of afferent activity will be detected only rarely. The spastic subject is therefore unable to differentiate low tension levels and probably is aware that he is above relaxation only when the experimenter says 'now'. When asked to repeat such tensions, the spastic subject produces the lowest level of activity that he can detect and so overshoots the target tension level. Even if this analysis is correct, subjects should be able to achieve a successful rank order of those tension levels which are above threshold.

It has been noted already that spastic subjects may have no successful system for monitoring neuromuscular activity. If this is so, their poor performance on this task would be expected. It is interesting to note the relationship between the accuracy that subjects achieved and the cues which they report using, although caution must, of course, be observed when drawing conclusions from these data. It is interesting to note that the most inaccurate subjects were those who reported using only wrist cues. Such information would not enable them to distinguish between changes which were produced by activity in the fore-arm flexors and changes which were produced when other muscle groups were contracted. Activity in related muscle groups is likely to occur in the spastic syndrome, therefore effort cues would be needed in order to differentiate changes in fore-arm flexor contraction.

The spastic subjects were observed to be less good at holding tension levels constant and they took longer to relax. These observations were supported by later investigations (see Chapter 7). It is therefore possible that the spastic subjects had a poorer opportunity to encode a tension level. They were also forced to wait longer before they were able to repeat the tension level and so may have forgotten more of its characteristics. In later studies these problems were overcome to some extent, but normal repetition accuracy was still not observed (Harrison 1973). It was concluded that the poor performance of the spastic subjects could not be accounted for totally by the problems which they have in holding tension levels and in achieving relaxation.

Another possible explanation for the poor performance shown by the spastic subjects is that they lack a suitable schema for encoding the tension level which is experienced. The subject is able to adjust activity in the muscle group and he is able to monitor afferent signals, but he is unable to classify the tension level which he is experiencing. An analogy can be drawn between the performance shown by normal and spastic subjects in the present experiment and that shown by musically trained and musically untrained persons who are asked to remember and match musical notes. The musically trained subject is able to classify the note when he first hears it, and this description will include all the features he must look for in the matching note. In contrast, the musically untrained subject has no such schema. He must try to define the variables which distinguish musical notes and he must try to develop a schema for describing the level of each variable which is present in a given note. Improved matching is likely to follow if he is given longer to code the note and if the experimenter reduces the delay before the matching is attempted. However these moves are unlikely to help the musically untrained subject to develop a system of classification which is as effective as that used by the musically trained subject. If spastic subjects lack a schema for encoding muscular activity, poor accuracy in repetition will persist even when relaxation and holding have been normalised. The next study was designed to investigate the system used by spastic subjects to code muscular activity.

Scaling is a tool which may be used to investigate how a person classifies a continuum. The procedure that was adopted in the present studies is known as the 'method of equally-appearing intervals'. This requires the subject to identify the levels of a variable which correspond to equally-spaced points on his subjective scale. This procedure can be illustrated by a study in which subjects are asked to classify different decibel levels in terms of subjective loudness. The subject is given a reference decibel level which he is told corresponds to five units of loudness. The task for the subject is to adjust the decibel level until it represents one unit of loudness, two units of loudness, three units of loudness, *etc.*

Figure 6 shows three different scales which might be produced. Scale A bears a linear relationship with the objective units (decibels) used to measure loudness. A logarithmic relationship is shown for Scale B. This indicates that the stimulus was judged to get louder when the decibel level was increased. Scale B also reveals that the subject was most sensitive to changes in decibel level at the bottom end of the range. The increase in decibel level which was needed to alter the assessment of loudness from one unit to two units was smaller than was required to alter the subjective assessment of loudness from four to five units. Scale C indicates that subjective assessment of loudness did not increase systematically when the decibel level was raised, *i.e.* the subject lacked an appropriate, subjective index of loudness. If these subjects were set the task of producing particular levels of loudness and their performance was scored in decibel units, subject A is likely to perform more accurately than subject B. Subject A will evaluate errors in a way which is consistent with the performance measure that is being applied. In contrast, subject B is likely to be unnecessarily precise in adjusting low levels of loudness and he is likely to incur large errors when he attempts to produce high levels. The subjective scale which was produced by subject B indicates that he is using cues which are appropriate for judging loudness. His task performance will therefore improve if he can learn to reclassify them in terms of the decibel scale. One way of helping him to do this is to provide him with augmented feedback which indicates changes in loudness in decibel units. Augmented feedback may help subject C to develop a concept of loudness and to identify inherent cues which signal changes in decibel level.

A comparison between the subjective scales used by normal and spastic subjects to classify neuromuscular activity will indicate whether these subjects differ in their ability to classify this continuum and it will also indicate whether the two groups are likely to differ in their sensitivity to changes in neuromuscular activity.

Experiment 1: The scaling of muscular activity by neurologically normal subjects

Procedure

Five university undergraduates took part in this study, with age range from 19 to 21 years. Surface electrodes were attached to record activity in the fore-arm flexor muscle group. Subjects were helped to isolate these muscles and to contract and relax them. The sensitivity of the apparatus was adjusted so that the reliable maximum contraction that a subject was able to produce occupied eight EMG units of the recording paper (Fig. 1). A copy of Fig. 7 was placed in front of the subject and the following instructions were given.

"Now that you have learned to tense up and relax the flexor muscle in your fore-arm, I want to discover how you conceptualise activity within it. In order to do this, I want you to picture a scale of tensions running from 0 to 7. Zero represents complete relaxation and 7 is a high level of tension which I will define for you. Having anchored points 0 and 7, I would like you to divide this range into seven equal parts so that the difference between 0 and 1 is the same as that between 1 and 2, 2 and 3, 3 and 4, 4 and 5, 5 and 6, 6 and 7. Having identified levels 0 and 7, I will ask you to produce each point on the scale. For example, when I say 'four', you should tense up from 0 to that tension which you think is 4, and when you reach it you should say 'now'. I shall then ask you to relax. When you have relaxed back down to 0, I will give you the number of the next tension that I want you to produce."

These instructions were expanded upon until the subject was certain that he understood exactly what he was being asked to do. The first stage was to give him a definition of points 0 to 7. On three occasions he was asked to tense up. When level 7 was reached the experimenter said 'now' and the subject relaxed down to 0. At the beginning of each of the five trials, two more definitions of 0 and 7 were given. Five

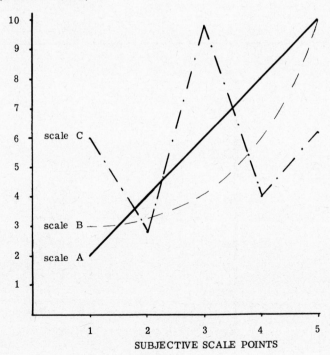

Fig. 6. Subjective scales of loudness.

61

trials followed in which the subject was asked to produce all of the seven points in randomised order. It was stressed to the subject that he should aim for equal intervals in his scale.

Results

The EMG records were scored in exactly the same way as outlined in the previous experiment. The mean muscular activity levels (EMG units) which were produced to represent the seven scale points are shown in Table I. These data were assessed in two ways. Spearman's Rank Correlation Coefficient (rs) was applied to assess whether subjective ranking correlated significantly with the rank order of the integrated EMG voltages, and Pearson's Coefficient of Correlation (R) was applied to assess whether intervals in the subjective evaluation of muscular activity reflected intervals in the integrated EMG scale.

TABLE I

The mean levels of integrated EMG activity produced as equivalent to the seven scale points set in Experiment 1

Subject	Scale Points							rs score	R score
	1	*2*	*3*	*4*	*5*	*6*	*7*		
N1	1.8	2.4	4.0	4.8	5.3	5.2	6.5	0.96, p<0.01	0.97, p<0.002
N2	0.9	1.8	1.6	2.4	2.8	5.5	7.0	0.96, p<0.01	0.92, p<0.01
N3	0.6	1.1	1.6	2.6	2.8	5.4	8.3	1.00, p<0.01	0.93, p<0.01
N4	1.6	2.2	3.9	2.8	4.7	6.6	7.0	0.96, p<0.01	0.98, p<0.001
N5	2.7	3.8	4.6	5.9	5.4	7.2	7.9	0.96, p<0.01	0.98, p<0.001

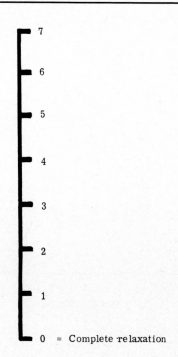

Fig. 7. The scaling guide.

Discussion

The scales produced by the neurologically normal subjects indicate that their ranking of muscular activity accorded with the integrated voltage EMG. It would have been surprising if this had not been so, for the integrated EMG is a very general measure of muscular activity. However there was no *a priori* reason for supposing that the integrated EMG would accord so exactly with subjective assessment of muscular activity. It is not clear whether the significant coefficients of correlation (R) are found because the integrated EMG mirrors the natural schema for classifying muscular activity or whether this occurs because the subjects have learned to conceptualise muscular activity using a scheme which correlates highly with EMG activity (Warren and Warren 1963, Treisman 1964).

Experiment 2: The scaling of muscular activity by spastic subjects

Procedure

Five spastic subjects took part in this experiment. The procedure was exactly the same as that outlined in Experiment 1 except that a six-point scale was introduced: in the previous experiment the subjects felt that the task was made difficult because there was no median scale point, and so the six-point scale was adopted to simplify the task. The apparatus was adjusted so that the reliable maximum contraction which a subject was able to produce occupied seven EMG units of the recording paper. The results achieved by the spastic subjects are given in Table II.

TABLE II

The mean levels of integrated EMG activity produced as equivalent to the six scale points set in Experiment 2

Subject	Scale Points						rs score	R score
	1	*2*	*3*	*4*	*5*	*6*		
Sp 1	4.8	4.0	3.9	4.6	4.0	4.6	-0.09, $p > 0.05$	-0.04, $p > 0.05$
Sp 2	1.6	1.5	2.7	2.8	2.2	5.4	0.77, $p > 0.05$	0.79, $p > 0.05$
Sp 3	3.7	4.3	4.7	4.4	4.6	6.8	0.83, $p < 0.05$	0.81, $p > 0.05$
Sp 4	0.7	1.0	1.6	2.8	3.5	5.9	1.00, $p < 0.01$	0.95, $p < 0.01$
Sp 5	1.1	1.8	2.8	3.2	3.8	5.8	1.00, $p < 0.01$	0.97, $p < 0.002$

Discussion

The results indicate that only three of the spastic subjects subjectively rank ordered muscular activity in accord with the integrated EMG scale. The integrated EMG is a very general measure of muscular activity and so it is difficult to imagine any useful system for classifying muscular activity which does not bear a significant rank correlation with it. A non-significant rs score may therefore be taken to indicate that the subject was unable to achieve an appropriate assessment of activity in the relevant muscle group. Only two of the spastic subjects achieved significant R scores.

Subjects were asked to measure muscular activity on a scale that had equal intervals. The different amounts of EMG activity found in successive scale intervals are therefore assumed to be perceptually equivalent. For each subject, an assessment was made of the increase in EMG activity which was required to bring about the shift from a given subjective scale point to the next. The data for the two subject groups are given in Fig. 8. Some points of caution must be noted before these data are interpreted. The assessments for the two spastic subjects who were unable to produce an appropriately-ranked set of muscular activity levels have been included. An inspection of Table II suggests that this is likely to have caused the amount of EMG activity encompassed by various scale intervals to be underestimated. Sp1, for example, produced roughly the same level of EMG voltage to represent each of the scale points: the difference in EMG activity between adjacent scale points is therefore small. It is important to note that the spastic subjects used only six scale intervals, whilst the neurologically normal subjects used seven. When subjects are asked to scale a given range of EMG activity the amount of activity assigned to a given scale interval will depend on the total number of scale intervals available. The fact that fewer scale points were used by the spastic subjects would account for less than a three per cent increase in the average amount of EMG activity which was assigned to any scale interval ($1/42 \times 100$ per cent). Spastic subjects are also likely to have had a smaller range of EMG activity to partition.

The amount of integrated EMG activity which was produced to represent scale point 1 was greater for the spastic subjects than for the normal subject group. The performance of Sp1 contributed greatly to this difference (Table II). However, even Sp3, who achieved a significant rs score, used a very high level of EMG activity to signify scale point 1. The amount of activity that is used to represent this point is a combination of the activity which is produced before the perceptual threshold is reached and the activity which is produced after this point and which signifies one unit of muscular activity. If Weber's Law applies, the amount of EMG activity that is required to move from threshold to scale point 1 is less than that required to move from scale point 1 to scale point 2. Figure 8 would therefore indicate that spastic subjects have an abnormally high threshold for detecting muscular activity. In the scales produced by the spastic subjects, a large range of EMG activity is bounded by scale points 5 and 6; this suggests that they will be inaccurate when judging high levels of muscular activity. These conclusions are consistent with the responses which were produced by spastic subjects when they were asked to repeat levels of neuromuscular activity. The spastic subjects did not appear to have any special difficulties in following the scaling procedure. The requirements to hold tension levels constant and to relax quickly, which they had found so difficult in the tension repetition task, were excluded. The inability of some spastic subjects to produce a suitably ranked set of responses in the scaling task is therefore taken to indicate a real lack of neuromuscular control.

In the scaling procedure, spastic subjects had to produce levels of neuromuscular activity in order to indicate the system of classification which they were using. The possibility therefore exists that spastic subjects do evaluate muscular activity with normal accuracy, but are unable to demonstrate this fact because they cannot produce precise levels of muscular activity. This possibility may be investigated by asking spastic subjects to label levels of induced muscular activity, although a major

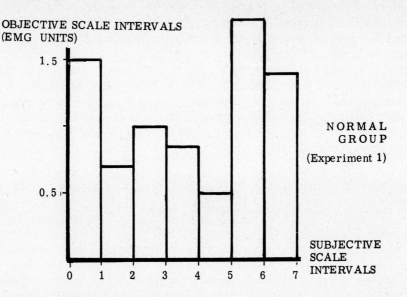

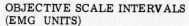

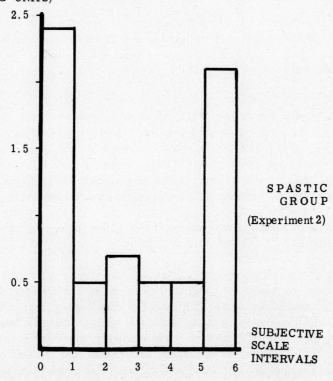

Fig. 8. The increments in neuromuscular activity judged to produce an equi-interval scale by the neurologically normal and spastic subject groups.

65

problem with this approach is that induced activity may differ from voluntary activity in critical ways. A second approach would be to ask subjects to label ongoing muscular activity, yet this again would favour the subject who is able to increase activity in a systematic fashion and who can hold the tension that he is being asked to classify. Although it is possible in theory to differentiate the ability to evaluate movements and the ability to control movements, it is questionable whether these do develop separately. The fact that a person is able to produce a contraction reliably implies that he has accurate motor control and that he is able to judge accurately when errors occur.

Experiment 3: A reassessment of the ability of spastic subjects to scale muscular activity

Procedure

During one tension repetition experiment, spastic subjects were provided with a meter display of integrated EMG activity in order to help them code the target tension levels. Some improvement was observed in the accuracy with which they repeated the tension levels that were set, although normal accuracy was not achieved (Harrison 1973). The meter indicated the level of integrated EMG activity which the subject was producing.

The present experiment was undertaken to assess whether any subjects had used this opportunity to acquire an appropriate system for assessing muscular activity or to re-code their existing scale in terms of the integrated EMG units. The data from the reassessments are given in Table III.

Discussion

It is clear from Tables II and III that some improvement in scaling ability was achieved after the subject had worked with the augmented feedback. Subject Sp2, who was previously unable to achieve a significant rs score, produced a perfectly ranked set of muscular activity levels. The augmented feedback helped her to isolate muscle signals which could be used to assess muscular activity appropriately. Subjects Sp2 and Sp3 acquired significant R scores in the present assessment.

Experiment 4: A second reassessment of the ability of spastic subjects to scale muscular activity

Procedure

The spastic subjects took part in the present experiment after they had completed a training programme, during which they learned to produce three levels of integrated EMG activity with stringent accuracy (Experiment 1, Chapter 7). During training, the levels of EMG activity were represented by a colour code and the subject was given no indication that the colours represented one, four and six EMG units. The subject knew the rank order of these levels of muscular activity but he was given no indication of how they should be classified on an interval scale. The results from this assessment are shown in Table IV.

TABLE III

The mean levels of integrated EMG activity produced as equivalent to the six scale points set in Experiment 3

Subject	Scale Points						rs score	R score
	1	*2*	*3*	*4*	*5*	*6*		
Sp 1	4.0	3.7	3.2	4.3	4.0	4.9	0.61, p>0.05	0.60, p>0.05
Sp 2	1.5	2.3	2.5	3.9	4.1	6.1	1.00, p<0.01	0.96, p<0.002
Sp 3	3.7	4.0	4.5	5.1	6.0	6.5	1.00, p<0.01	0.99, p<0.001
Sp 4	0.8	1.1	1.4	2.5	2.4	4.7	0.94, p<0.01	0.92, p<0.01
Sp 5	1.5	2.6	3.1	3.4	3.6	6.6	1.00, p<0.01	0.90, p<0.02

TABLE IV

The mean levels of integrated EMG activity produced as equivalent to the six scale points set in Experiment 4

Subject	Scale Points						rs score	R score
	1	*2*	*3*	*4*	*5*	*6*		
Sp 1	1.4	3.8	3.9	4.7	5.4	7.2	1.00, p<0.01	0.96, p<0.01
Sp 2	1.3	2.8	3.5	4.0	4.3	6.0	1.00, p<0.01	0.97, p<0.02
Sp 3	0.4	1.9	2.5	2.9	4.2	4.7	1.00, p<0.01	0.98, p<0.001
Sp 4	0.9	1.6	2.2	2.8	3.5	4.7	1.00, p<0.01	0.99, p<0.001
Sp 5	1.0	1.6	1.9	2.7	3.6	5.2	1.00, p<0.01	0.97, p<0.002

Discussion

The ability of spastic subjects to scale muscular activity improved after they participated in the training programme described above. All of the subjects produced a perfectly-ranked set of integrated EMG voltages. All five subjects achieved significant R scores. Only one subject (Sp3) showed an R score which was smaller than that achieved in Experiment 3. It has been stressed already that there is no reason why an efficient index of muscular activity should bear a significant coefficient of correlation (R) with the integrated EMG scale. The fact that normal subjects showed significant R scores and that spastic subjects acquired these after they had been trained to regulate muscular activity accurately suggests that the integrated EMG scale reflects the natural schema for judging muscular activity. If this is so, the integrated EMG is a very appropriate index of muscular activity. It should provide an excellent form of augmented feedback, for changes in the integrated EMG measure will correspond to the changes which are occurring in inherent signals.

During the training programme, the subjects learned to produce a low level of muscular activity accurately. In previous studies, spastic subjects were observed to have difficulty in regulating low tension levels and it was speculated that they had an abnormally high threshold for detecting muscular activity. In the present experiment, much smaller integrated EMG levels were produced to represent scale point 1. This suggests that the subjects had retained strategies which they had learned in the training programme for suppressing excess activity and for detecting changes in muscular activity at this level. This indicates that the improvements in motor control acquired during the training programme were not restricted to the three levels of muscular activity that were taught. A general improvement in the spastic subjects' ability to regulate and evaluate muscular activity is evidenced by their improved scaling performance. The scaling paradigm therefore proved useful for detecting changes in the subjects' ability to evaluate and control motor activity.

Induced Activity in the Spastic Neuromusculature

When the spastic person contracts a muscle, activity in related muscle groups may be produced. The present studies were designed to investigate whether the amount of activity which is induced by a given contraction is reliable or whether it varies from one occasion to the next. If it does vary, the spastic person will have greater difficulty in learning to programme and monitor movements accurately and in acquiring reliable strategies for suppressing unwanted muscular activity. The present experiments investigated the amount of activity produced in the fore-arm extensor muscle group when the spastic subject contracts the fore-arm flexor muscle group. Induced activity is likely to occur in the extensor group because it contains muscles which are antagonistic and synergistic to the flexor muscles. The task for the subject was to regulate fore-arm flexor activity. However, it has been argued already that one of the likely consequences of induced activity is that the spastic individual fails to learn to differentiate the motor neurons associated with particular muscle groups. If this is so, the spastic person is likely to fire extensor motor neurons when he is asked to contract the flexor muscles.

Activity in the two muscle groups was recorded during three experiments in which the ability of spastic subjects to repeat levels of muscular activity was being assessed. The first experiment was the one reported in this paper. The procedure followed in the second experiment was exactly the same: it served to reassess the accuracy achieved by the spastic subjects after they had been exposed to the integrated EMG scale of muscular activity (Harrison 1973). In the third experiment, the subject was provided with a meter which indicated the level of integrated EMG activity he was producing. The subject watched the meter while he attempted to identify the target tension level (Harrison *op. cit.*), then the meter was removed and the subject attempted to repeat the tension level that was set. The data from all three experiments have been included in order to increase the likelihood of detecting any variations in induced activity.

The present study assessed the activity in the flexor and extensor muscles during the setting and repetition stages of these experiments. The purpose was to investigate whether the amount of extensor activity induced by a given flexor contraction remained constant.

Procedure

Surface electrodes were attached to record activity in the fore-arm flexor muscle group and the fore-arm extensor muscle group. Subjects were asked to ignore the set of electrodes placed over the extensor group and were not given any information which would help them to detect when the extensor group was active. Amplification in the channel recording extensor activity was set at the same level as that used for flexor activity. The procedure which was followed in the tension repetition experiments is outlined in an earlier section of this paper.

Results

The records were scored to provide the following data:

F.R. The level of flexor activity which represented the subject's attempt at repeating the target tension level.

E.R. The level of extensor activity which was concurrent with F.R.

E.S. The level of extensor activity that was present during the setting stage when the flexor group was producing the target tension level.

F.S. The target tension level of flexor activity.

The method which was developed to assess E.S. was as follows. First of all a distinction was drawn between those occasions during the setting stage when the subject held the F.S. level for one second or longer and those when the F.S. level was held for less than one second: the latter were termed 'cross-over points'. An assessment of E.S. was made for each cross-over point and for each period of holding For each cross-over point, the initial level of E.S. which occurred with F.S. was noted. Two assessments of E.S. were made for each one second period of holding: one was the level of extensor activity present after 400 msecs; the second was the level present after one second. The E.S. value that was used was the mean of the various assessments made.

Nine levels of F.S. were used and these were tested in each of five trials. Forty-five assessments of the flexor/extensor activity ratio were made for each subject during the setting stage, and 45 were made for the repetition stage. The data from five subjects were collected in each experiment.

The levels of extensor and flexor activity which were observed during the setting and repetition stages of an experiment are shown in Fig. 9. This indicates that increases in flexor activity were associated with increases in activity in the extensor muscle group. The same pattern of covariance was observed when the data for individual subjects were examined. A Spearman Rank Correlation Coefficient (rs) between flexor activity and extensor activity was significant for all of the subjects in each of the three experiments ($p < 0.05$). Figure 9 also suggests that the ratio between flexor and extensor activity did not vary between the setting and repetition stages; *i.e.* the F.S./E.S. ratio was the same as the F.R./E.R. ratio. The data in Fig. 9 is for the group: individuals may show variations which are lost when the group curves are computed and so the following analysis was developed in an attempt to overcome this problem.

The rationale underlying the test was as follows. If the ratio between extensor and flexor activity remains constant, a knowledge of the ratio at the setting stage and a knowledge of F.R. will be sufficient to enable one to predict E.R. accurately. If the predicted E.R. values (P.E.R.) differ significantly from the observed values of E.R., it follows that the extensor/flexor ratio has changed between the setting stage and the repetition stage. For each subject, 45 values of P.E.R. were computed. An assessment of the relationship between extensor and flexor activity was made using the 45 pairs of F.S. and E.S. scores which were measured. The exponential or linear equation which best described the relationship between extensor and flexor activity was computed. Given this equation, values of P.E.R. were computed for the 45 F.R. scores. An analysis of variance was used to compare the P.E.R. scores and the E.R. scores for each of the three experiments (Fig. 10). The P.E.R. scores and the E.R. scores did not differ significantly ($p > 0.05$).

Discussion

The results failed to show any significant change in the relationship between flexor activity and extensor activity in the setting and repetition stages of the experiment. With due regard to the logical impossibility of proving the Null Hypothesis, a constant relationship between activity in these two muscle groups is indicated. An inspection of the raw data accords with this view. Further studies are required to investigate whether the reliability shown is typical of other muscle groups. A number of important consequences follow if a contraction produces a reliable amount of induced activity. If induced activity varied, subjects would find it difficult to programme movements accurately and to acquire reliable strategies for suppressing unwanted activity. When induced activity can be predicted accurately, the individual is in a position to acquire a reliable definition of the functioning of his neuro-musculature.

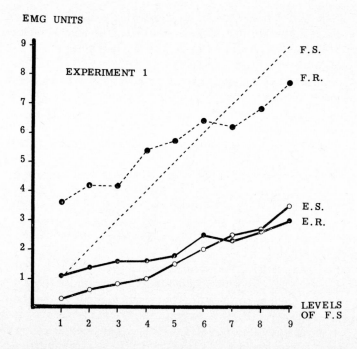

Fig. 9 (*and see facing page*). The relationships between fore-arm flexor and fore-arm extensor activity observed during the setting and repetition stages of three experiments performed by spastic subjects. (F.S., F.R., E.S. and E.R. are defined in the text.)

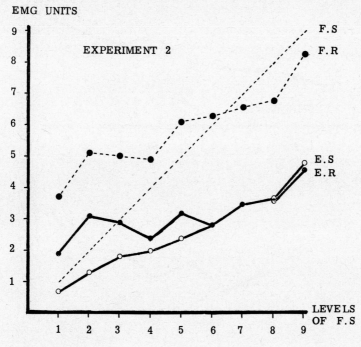

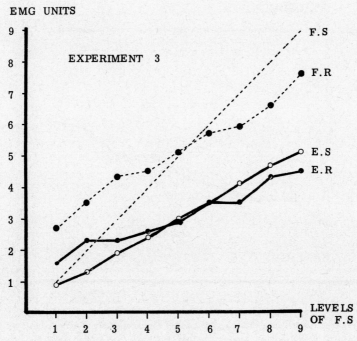

71

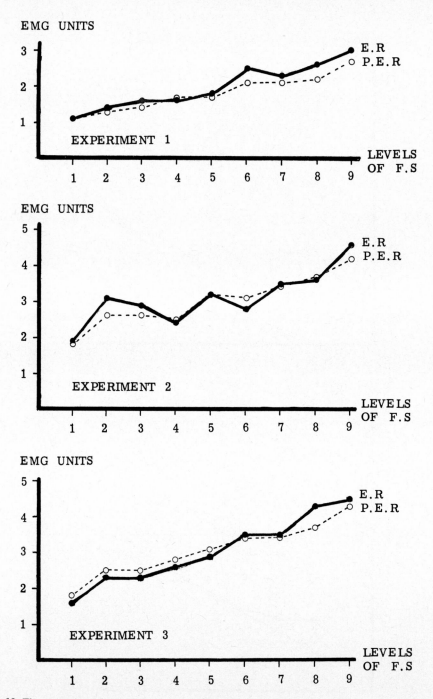

Fig. 10. The concordance between the levels of induced fore-arm extensor activity observed (E.R.) and those predicted on the assumption that induced activity is reliably produced in the spastic system (P.E.R., F.S., E.R. and P.E.R. are defined in the text.)

The experiment demonstrated that when the subject contracted the fore-arm flexor muscle group, a constant level of activity in the extensor group was produced. The very fact that this pattern is produced reliably may mean that the subject never learns to differentiate flexor activity. He may indeed encode the contractions he produces in terms of characteristics of the *pattern* of activity present, and not in terms of activity in any one muscle. If he adopts this system of classification, errors are likely to occur when he is called upon to repeat levels of activity in one of these muscles. Table V illustrates this point.

TABLE V

The levels of flexor and extensor activity present for eight hypothetical states of neuromuscular activity

States	1	2	3	4	5	6	7	8
Flexor activity	2	3	4	5	6	7	8	9
Induced extensor activity	1	1½	2	2⅓	3	3	5	7

If the subject chooses to code muscular activity in terms of the *ratio* of activity in the two muscle groups, States 1, 2, 3 and 5 will be perceptually indistinguishable for him. Therefore if he is set the task of repeating flexor level 2, he is likely to overshoot the target tension level. If he codes muscular activity in terms of the *difference* in activity between the two muscle groups, States 3 and 8 will be subjectively the same and he is likely to underestimate the target tension level when he is asked to repeat flexor level 9. These errors occur because the system used by the subject to judge whether a response is accurate is different from that used by the experimenter. It is important to try to assess whether the spastic subjects were in fact using such strategies to evaluate neuromuscular activity. That they were able to adjust muscular activity appropriately when asked to tense up or to relax suggests that very different levels of neuromuscular activity were not perceptually equivalent (as is required by the explanation offered above). An inspection of the polygraph records revealed that activity in the extensor group began after activity in the fore-arm flexors and that it did not occur when the flexor group was fully relaxed. These observations suggest that the spastic subjects were differentially firing flexor motor neurons and that they were not programming concurrent activity in the flexor and extensor muscles. It therefore appears unlikely that these subjects were using precise schema for coding the levels of neuromuscular activity which were to be repeated. A more probable explanation for their poor performance is that it is a reflection of their inability to evaluate and regulate fore-arm flexor activity accurately.

SUMMARY

The review of the components of neuromuscular control indicated the complexity of controls of movement which have to be acquired by all developing children, both normal and abnormal, and investigated the reasons why spastic individuals have difficulty in refining their motor performance.

The first experiments were designed to investigate the accuracy with which spastic individuals regulate and evaluate activity in a single muscle group. When asked to repeat specified levels of fore-arm flexor activity their performance was poor. Similar inaccuracy was shown when spastic subjects subjectively scaled neuromuscular activity. Taken together, these experiments demonstrate that spastic adults had failed to use their everyday experience to learn to control the simplest of movements with normal precision. The final experiment investigated the activity induced in the extensor muscle group when the flexor muscles are contracted. In this instance, although the spastic neuromusculature was functioning abnormally, it was found to be functioning reliably. This is an important prerequisite if the spastic individual is to achieve a reliable functional definition of his neuromusculature and reliable strategies for suppressing unwanted activity.

REFERENCES

Davis, J. F. (1952) *'Manual of Surface Electromyography.'* Laboratory for Psychological Studies, Allan Memorial Institute of Psychiatry, Montreal.
Harrison, A. (1973) 'Studies of neuromuscular control in spastic persons.' Unpublished Ph.D. thesis, Sheffield University.
Lenman, J. A. R., Ritchie, A. E. (1970) *Clinical Electromyography.* London: Pitman Medical.
Lippold, O. C. J. (1967) 'Electromyography.' *In* Venables, P. H., Martin, I. (Eds.) *A Manual of Psycho-physiological Methods.* Amsterdam: North-Holland; New York: Wiley.
Triesman, M. (1964) 'Sensory scaling and the psychophysical law.' *Quarterly Journal of Experimental Psychology,* **16,** 11.
Warren, R. M., Warren, R. P. (1963) 'A critique of S. S. Stevens' "New Psychophysics"'. *Perceptual and Motor Skills,* **16,** 797.

CHAPTER SEVEN

Training Spastic Individuals to Achieve Better Neuromuscular Control Using Electromyographic Feedback

ANN HARRISON

Neurologically normal persons develop movement control in the course of learning to perform everyday tasks more efficiently, but it is unlikely that the spastic individual will be able to realize his full potential for motor control under such conditions. Everyday tasks usually require complex patterns of movement and it is doubtful whether the spastic person possesses enough motor control to be able to alter his performance of them in any systematic fashion. Indeed, earlier experiments demonstrated that spastic adults were unable to regulate activity in one muscle group with normal precision (see Chapter 6).

The present studies investigated ways of helping spastic persons to achieve better neuromuscular control. The general procedure used was to ask the subjects to make very simple movements and to provide them with a clear assessment of how accurately they performed. This experience offers the spastic individual the opportunity of learning to construct appropriate movement programmes, of identifying suitable movement cues and of defining relevant sources of interference. A general improvement in motor control should be seen if the spastic subject is able to achieve a better functional definition of the interplay of reflex and voluntary activity in his neuromusculature. More normal accuracy should follow if he learns to suppress alpha motoneuron hyperactivity or to inhibit primitive and abnormal reflexes.

Harrison and Connolly (1971) showed that spastic individuals are able to learn to control fine levels of neuromuscular activity when they are provided with EMG feedback. The spastic subjects took a long time to reduce activity in the fore-arm flexor muscles to the level which was required. However, the control which they demonstrated in post-training sessions was equal to that achieved by the neurologically normal subjects who were tested. A similar method was used by Netsell and Cleeland (1973) to train a patient suffering from Parkinson's disease to reduce hyperactivity in the levator labii superioris muscle. Hyperactivity in this muscle was producing complete bilateral retraction of the upper lip. The patient was provided with augmented feedback in the form of a tone whose frequency varied with the EMG output from the relevant muscle: the patient's task was, therefore, to try to lower the frequency of the tone. After five half-hour sessions considerable improvement had been achieved.

In the first of the present experiments, subjects were given augmented feedback in the form of a meter display of EMG activity. The scaling experiments reported earlier suggest that the integrated EMG index will provide a particularly useful form of feedback because it should highlight inherent movement cues very effectively. An assessment was made of the benefits to be gained by providing such feedback when the spastic individual is asked to maintain neuromuscular activity at a prescribed level or to relax as quickly as possible. In later experiments, continuous feedback was not provided; instead, the subject was told at the end of each attempt at a task exactly how well he had performed. The subject should be able to use such knowledge of results to evaluate various ways of tackling a task and to experiment with strategies for refining his performance. This system was used in an attempt to train spastic persons to produce accurate levels of activity in the flexor and biceps muscles of the fore-arm. The relative advantages of using knowledge of results and continuous augmented feedback will be discussed later.

RELAXATION

The present experiments compared the time taken by spastic and neurologically normal persons to reduce neuromuscular activity and to achieve the complete relaxation of a muscle. The speed with which this is achieved reflects the accuracy with which a person is able to detect and to regulate neuromuscular activity. A special difficulty facing the spastic individual is that of defining the cause of any residual activity, for many types of voluntary and reflex firings might be responsible. Earlier experiments indicated that spastic persons have difficulty in evaluating and controlling muscular activity. It is therefore likely that spastic persons will take longer to achieve complete relaxation.

Experiment 1: An assessment of the time taken by neurologically normal and spastic persons to achieve relaxation of the fore-arm flexors

Procedure

Five university undergraduates whose ages ranged from 18 to 20 years took part in this study; none of them had any known neurological abnormality. Five spastic individuals, ranging in age from 19 to 30 years, also took part. The neurologically normal subjects used their non-dominant arm; spastic subjects used their more impaired limb.

The general procedure that was outlined earlier in Chapter 6 was again followed. Surface electrodes were attached to record activity from the fore-arm flexor muscle group. The experimenter helped the subject to identify the relevant muscles and to find an arm posture which allowed complete relaxation of the fore-arm flexors to be achieved. The sensitivity of the apparatus was adjusted so that the reliable maximum contraction which a subject was able to produce occupied 10 EMG units of the polygraph record (Fig. 1). The times taken by a subject to relax from tension levels 1 to 9 were measured. Five trials were completed; each contained all nine tension levels in randomised order. A preliminary trial, in which tension levels 1 and 9 were tested, was introduced to give the subject an opportunity to practise the procedure. Each tension level was tested in the following way. The subject was told that he should tense up gradually. When the relevant tension level was reached, the experimenter said 'now' and the subject relaxed as quickly as he could. A mark was made on the permanent record when the experimenter said 'now'. When complete relaxation was achieved, the next tension level was tested. A short rest was taken at the end of each trial.

Results

The polygraph records were scored to provide an assessment of the time taken to achieve complete relaxation (Fig. 1). A paper speed of five mm per sec had been used, each vertical mm division therefore represented 0.2 sec (one *time unit*). The record division that preceded the 'now' instruction was defined as the start of relaxation. The number of complete record divisions (time units) which occurred before baseline activity was regained was computed. Figure 2 compares the relaxation times produced by the two subject groups. An analysis of variance was applied to these data; this indicated that the spastic subjects took significantly longer to achieve complete relaxation ($F = 39.25$; $df = 1,8$; $p < 0.001$). The five trials did not differ significantly ($p > 0.05$) nor did the nine tension levels. No significant interactions were found.

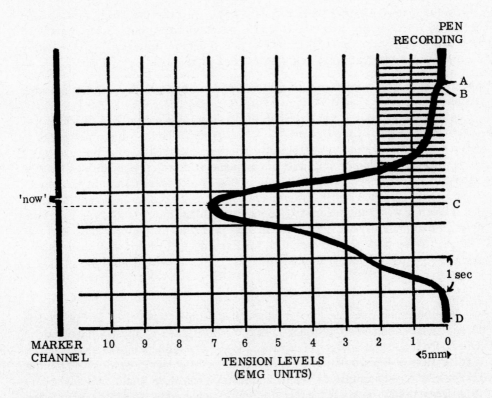

Fig. 1. The method used to compute relaxation times in Experiments 1 and 2. (D—subject asked to tense up, C—defined as beginning of relaxation period, A—point when baseline regained, B—defined as termination of relaxation.) Operationally defined relaxation time equals AC (17 time units, 3.4 seconds).

77

Discussion

The experiment demonstrated that the spastic individuals took approximately six times longer to achieve relaxation than the neurologically normal subjects who were tested. The polygraph records indicate that subjects quickly relaxed to a level just above baseline and spent the majority of time eliminating the low level of activity which remained. On the basis of the scaling experiments which were reported earlier, it is likely that subjects had difficulty detecting these low levels of neuro-muscular activity and it is probable that some were sub-threshold. When operating at sub-threshold levels, a subject would be unable to evaluate accurately whether the strategy he was employing to reduce activity was successful or not. The wastefulness of a trial-and-error search may account for the disproportionately long time taken to eliminate the residual activity.

The fact that the spastic subjects were able to complete the task indicates that they did have strategies for reducing neuromuscular activity. The longer time taken by these subjects may be accounted for in terms of a heightened threshold for detecting neuromuscular activity, the difficulties which they have when evaluating and regulating neuromuscular activity or the problems which they face in identifying the cause of any residual activity.

In the following experiment, a meter display was provided which indicated the integrated EMG output from the fore-arm flexor muscle group. Such augmented feedback should help the subject to evaluate different strategies for eliminating neuromuscular activity and so help him to relax more quickly.

Experiment 2: The performance of spastic subjects when provided with augmented feedback

Augmented feedback was provided in the form of a meter (Fig. 3) which was driven by the output of the Devices AC8 preamplifier. The inertia characteristics of the meter pointer and the pens of the polygraph were matched, so that the reading on the meter mirrored that produced on the permanent record. The ten divisions on the meter dial corresponded to the ten tension levels which were tested. Subjects were briefed until they were clear that movements of the meter pen towards zero indicated that relaxation was being successfully achieved and that movements away from zero signified that muscular activity was being increased. The testing procedure that was followed was the same as that described for Experiment 1 except that subjects were required to watch the meter throughout.

Results

The relaxation times achieved by the spastic subjects are given in Fig. 2. The introduction of augmented feedback halved the time taken by spastic individuals to achieve relaxation. An analysis of variance showed this reduction to be significant (F = 10.16; df = 1,4; $p < 0.05$). The five trials did not differ significantly ($p > 0.05$) nor did the nine tension levels; no significant interactions were found. An analysis of variance was used to compare the relaxation times achieved by the spastic group when using augmented feedback with those produced by the neurologically normal subjects working without the meter. This analysis showed that the spastic subjects were still significantly slower (F = 9.00; df = 1,8; p < 0.05) despite the great improvement in their performance.

Discussion

The ability of spastic individuals to achieve fore-arm flexor relaxation was significantly improved in the second experiment. This improvement was not attributed to the fact that subjects were performing the task for a second time because no practice effects were shown in the individual experiments. Instead, it was presumed to be caused by the introduction of an unambiguous index of neuromuscular activity

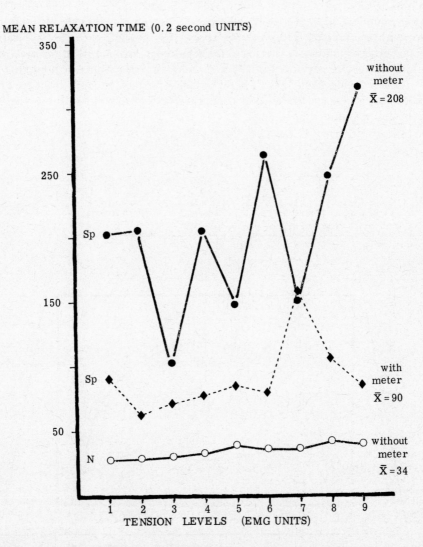

Fig. 2. The relaxation times achieved by the neurologically normal (N) and spastic (Sp) subject groups in Experiments 1 and 2.

which enabled subjects to select successful strategies for reducing fore-arm flexor activity. No post-training testing sessions were included and so it is not known whether faster relaxation times were retained when the augmented feedback was removed. A permanent improvement in performance would depend on the spastic individuals being able to isolate movement cues which would enable them to assess low levels of contraction. The findings of the last experiments reported in this paper indicate that this is possible.

The relaxation times produced by the spastic individuals in the present experiment were still abnormally slow. These subjects did not experience a long training session with the augmented feedback and so it is possible that further improvement would be achieved with an extended period, though no trend in this direction was observed across the five trials. It is possible that once subjects had isolated generally successful strategies for achieving relaxation, then the requirement to watch the meter may have actually impeded their performance by preventing their full attention being given to the task. The major point to be made from the present findings is that the spastic subjects demonstrated that they do have a potential for better motor control.

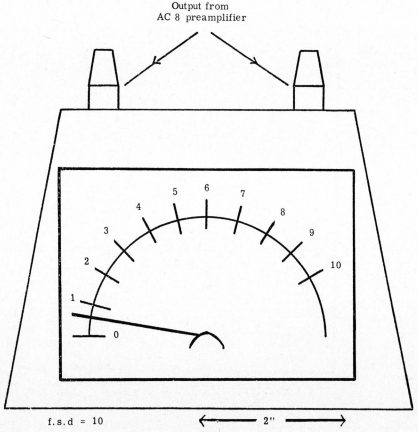

Fig. 3. The voltmeter used to provide augmented feedback in Experiments 2 and 4.

The present experiments investigated the performance of neurologically normal and spastic individuals when they are asked to maintain specific levels of neuro-muscular activity. Accuracy depends upon the person being capable of detecting shifts away from the prescribed level and of appropriately altering activity in the relevant muscle. An individual's performance will be marred if he is unable to evaluate and regulate neuromuscular activity accurately. The same groups of subjects were employed in the relaxation and tension maintenance studies. The relaxation studies were completed first because the tension maintenance tasks also required subjects to achieve complete relaxation. The experiments were tackled in the order 1, 3, 2 and 4. A day's rest was taken between Experiments 3 and 2.

Experiment 3: The accuracy shown by neurologically normal and spastic persons when they are asked to maintain particular levels of fore-arm flexor activity

Procedure

The initial procedure was identical with that described for Experiment 1. Subjects were told that the purpose of the experiment was to assess how accurately they were able to maintain particular levels of fore-arm flexor activity. A practice trial, during which tension levels 1 and 9 were tested, was used to familiarise a subject with the procedure. Subjects were asked to tense up in a controlled way, gradually enough to have a clear idea of the tension level that was to be held, but not so slowly that they would fail to reach the higher levels when these were set. The following instructions were used.

"At some point whilst you are tensing up I shall say 'hold'; at this command you should maintain the current tension as accurately as you can for ten seconds. You should make any compensations which you feel are necessary during these ten seconds, tensing up if you feel that the muscle has become too relaxed, and relaxing if you think that the muscle has become more tense."

At the end of the ten-second holding period, the subject was asked to relax completely. When complete relaxation was achieved, the next tension level was tested. Five trials were given, each contained all nine tension levels in randomised order. A short rest was taken at the end of each trial.

Results

The polygraph records were scored to provide an assessment of task performance (Fig. 4). The vertical record division that preceded the 'hold' marker was defined as the start of the holding period. The integrated EMG activity levels which were present at the ten one-second intervals (5 mm) beyond this point were computed. Neuromuscular activity levels were measured with an accuracy of 0.2 EMG units; each score was rounded in the direction of least error. The mean of the ten scores for each holding period provides an assessment of the appropriateness of the activity levels produced. Figure 5 compares the mean neuromuscular activity levels produced by the spastic and normal subject groups. This indicates that a more restricted range of tension levels was produced by the spastic subjects and that these were less appropriate to the levels which had been designated than those generated by the neurologically normal individuals. An analysis of variance was used to evaluate these differences; the subject group/tension level interaction was found to be highly significant (F = 7.81; df = 8,64; p < 0.001).

A second assessment of the accuracy shown when subjects were asked to maintain a particular level of neuromuscular activity was achieved by tracing the changes in activity which occurred during the ten-second holding period (Fig. 6). Subjects typically overshot the designated neuromuscular activity level. After this, the neurologically normal subjects managed to maintain this level accurately and showed very little deviation. In contrast, the spastic subjects failed to check a gradual loss of neuromuscular activity during the remainder of the holding period. An analysis of variance confirmed that the two subject groups performed differently; the subject group/holding period interaction was highly significant (F = 4.85; df = 10.80; p < 0.001).

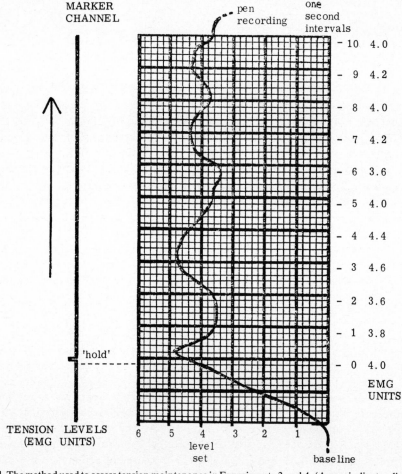

Fig. 4. The method used to assess tension maintenance in Experiments 3 and 4. (Arrow indicates direction of recording.)

Discussion

The results showed that spastic individuals are less able to maintain specified levels of neuromuscular activity. They exhibited a less accurate appreciation of the target neuromuscular activity levels and a poor ability to compensate for deviations away from the levels which they had chosen to hold. The initial overshooting of a target tension was shown by both subject groups and it is probably due to the fact that subjects were still tensing up when the instruction to hold was given. It is therefore likely that they had an inflated evaluation of the target neuromuscular activity level. The normal subjects showed little deviation from the level which they chose to hold, whilst the spastic individuals drifted further and further from it. It is not clear from this experiment whether spastic individuals failed to detect these changes in neuromuscular activity or whether they were unable to find successful methods for making the corrections which they knew to be necessary. The performance of these subjects in the next experiment, when they were provided with augmented feedback, should clarify this issue.

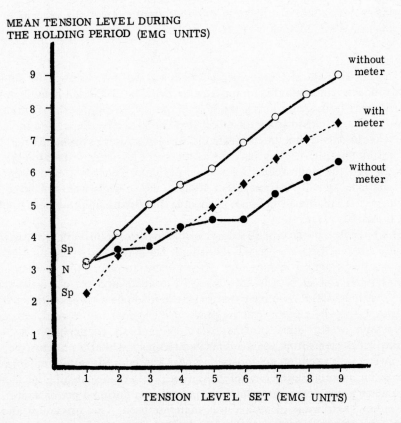

Fig. 5. The accuracy of tension maintenance displayed by the neurologically normal (N) and spastic (Sp) subject groups in Experiments 3 and 4.

83

Experiment 4: The performance of spastic subjects when provided with augmented feedback

The meter described in Experiment 2 was used to provide the subjects with augmented feedback. The testing procedure was the same as that outlined above except that subjects were required to watch the meter display throughout.

Results

The performances produced by the spastic individuals when working with and without augmented feedback are shown in Figs. 5 and 6. When subjects used the meter the mean levels of neuromuscular activity which they produced during the holding periods became more appropriate. An analysis of variance showed this improvement to be significant ($F = 2.42$; $df = 8,32$; $p < 0.05$). The levels produced in Experiment 4 no longer differed significantly ($p > 0.05$) from those produced by the neurologically normal subjects who took part in Experiment 3. Some improvement in the spastic individuals' ability to control drift during the holding period was also observed, particularly in the latter seconds. However, this improvement was not great enough to reach significance ($p > 0.05$) and the performance of the spastic subjects on Experiment 4 was still significantly different from that of the normal group in Experiment 3 ($F = 2.04$; $df = 10,80$; $p < 0.05$).

Discussion

The introduction of the augmented feedback did help the spastic subjects to identify the relevant levels of neuromuscular activity, but it did not help them to curb the drift away from these during the holding period, except, perhaps, towards the end. The spastic individuals understood that the meter readings were indicating a gradual loss of activity, but they were unable to isolate strategies to counter these drifts. It is possible that the holding period was too short for them to isolate appropriate methods, and the improvement shown in the latter seconds would support this interpretation. As with the relaxation studies, the subjects were not given a long training period with the meter and it is possible that further improvement would take place if this was extended.

It is possible that the normal subject is able to perform this task in a way which is radically different from the spastic individual. He may have set his neuromuscular system so that changes in muscular activity were automatically compensated for (Phillips 1969) and so he was not having to evaluate and correct neuromuscular activity continuously. It is unlikely that spastic individuals would acquire such skilful strategies during the present training procedure because they worked with any one level for only a short time and they were continuously changing levels. Another difficulty which stems from using augmented feedback is that it prevents the subject from giving full attention to inherent movement cues. It also probably places emphasis on making continuous compensation rather than searching for movement programmes which demand the minimum of revision during a performance. In the next studies, 'knowledge of results' was therefore used. This procedure allows the subject to give his full attention to inherent movement cues and prevents him from becoming reliant upon additional information for judging what corrections are required.

Experiment 5: Training spastic individuals to produce levels of fore-arm activity accurately

This experiment investigated whether spastic individuals are able to learn to produce low, intermediate and high levels of neuromuscular activity with stringent accuracy. The general procedure was simple: a subject was asked to try to produce a particular level of fore-arm flexor contraction; after each attempt, he was told whether it was too high, too low or correct. More detailed feedback in terms of size of error was not given because it was not certain that this could be meaningful to the subject. In theory, the knowledge of results should enable the subject to isolate successful movement programmes, accurate movement cues and to detect sources of interference. Harrison and Connolly (1971) demonstrated that spastic individuals are able to learn to control very fine levels of neuromuscular activity. The present experiment investigated whether they have a potential for producing a full range of activity levels with normal precision.

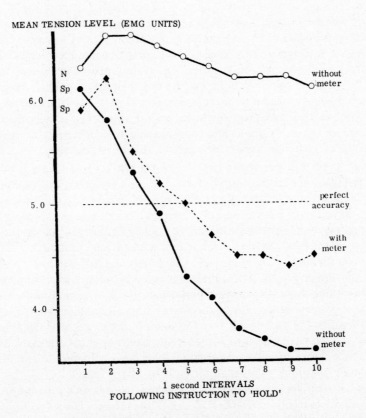

Fig. 6. The progress of tension maintenance observed during the holding period for the neurologically normal (N) and spastic (Sp) subject groups in Experiments 3 and 4.

Procedure

The general procedure which was followed was the same as that described for Experiment 1. Five spastic persons took part in this study. Each subject used his more severely impaired limb throughout training. The training programme consisted of the eight sections that are outlined below.

SECTION 1. The experimenter helped a subject to identify the fore-arm flexor muscles. The subject was told to avoid movements of the head, upper arm and opposite arm and to avoid intrinsic movements of the hand. The sensitivity of the apparatus was adjusted until the reliable maximum contraction which a subject was able to produce occupied seven EMG units of the recording paper (Fig. 7). A subject was set the task of learning to produce six, four and one EMG units, which were called the 'Black', 'Red' and 'White' targets respectively. His attempts were measured with an accuracy of 0.2 EMG units; scores were rounded in the direction of least error. An accurate performance was defined as one which was within the band of ± 0.2 EMG units of the target level. For example, a correct response for the Black target lay within the range 5.81 to 6.19 EMG units.

SECTION 2. The purpose of this section was to evaluate the subject's initial ability to produce the target tension levels. The subject was given a copy of Fig. 8 and he was told that three tension levels were to be tested, of which Black was the highest, White the lowest and Red an intermediate level. His initial control was assessed by asking him to repeat the target activity levels. Five trials were completed; each contained the three target levels in randomised order. The testing procedure was as follows. The subject was told the colour to be tested; he was then asked to tense up gradually so that he would gain a clear idea of the level that was to be aimed for. When the target activity level was reached, the experimenter said 'now'. The subject then relaxed as quickly as he could. When complete relaxation was achieved, he was asked to produce the target tension level. He signified this by saying 'now'.

SECTION 3. In this section, subjects were trained to produce each of the target activity levels accurately; the order in which these were taken was randomised. The procedure for each target was as follows. The subject was first told the colour he was to learn and was given a rough idea of the target level by asking him twice to tense up and saying 'now' when the target level was reached. After this, the subject tensed up until he thought that the target level was reached and said 'now'. A mark was produced on the permanent record and the subject was told whether his attempt was too high, too low or correct. The subject continued to produce levels until he managed to produce three successive correct performances. Rest periods were taken when subject or experimenter thought they were necessary. Immediately following his three correct attempts, the subject was asked to produce the target level five times. During this recall test, no feedback was given as to the accuracy of his attempts. This section was complete when criterion performance had been achieved for all three target activity levels and immediate recall for each had been tested.

SECTION 4. This section followed the previous one immediately and it tested the subject's ability to recall the Black, Red and White targets. The subject was reminded that the Black level was the highest, White the lowest and Red an intermediate level. He was given no feedback as to the accuracy of his attempts. Five trials were

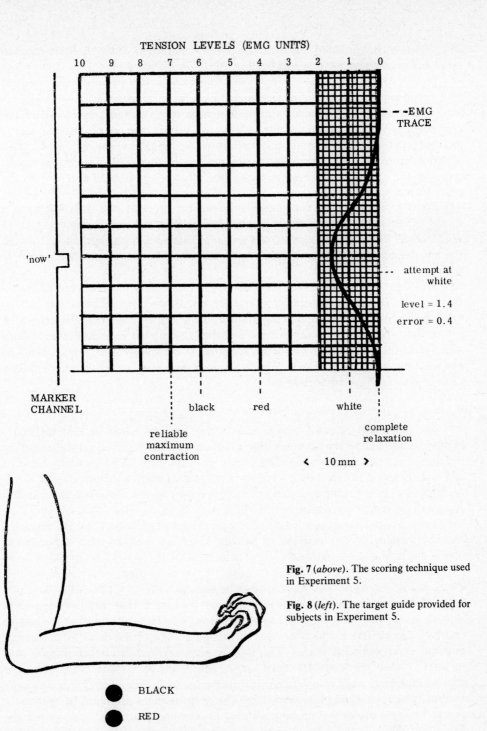

Fig. 7 (*above*). The scoring technique used in Experiment 5.

Fig. 8 (*left*). The target guide provided for subjects in Experiment 5.

87

completed; each contained all three targets in randomised order. A short rest was taken before the next section was begun.

SECTION 5. In this section, subjects were trained to switch from one target to the next, producing each of them accurately. Lists were prepared that consisted of blocks, each of which contained the three tension levels in randomised order. The experimenter worked through a list, telling the subject the colour that he was to produce and telling him whether his attempt was too high, too low, or correct. This continued until the subject managed to produce two successive blocks accurately, *i.e.,* six successive accurate target levels. Rests were taken when thought necessary by the experimenter or subject.

SECTION 6. This section immediately followed the previous one. It consisted of a repeat of Section 4. A short rest was taken before Section 7 was begun.

SECTION 7. This section consisted of a repeat of Section 5; it was introduced to bring the subject back to criterion accuracy when switching from one target level to another.

SECTION 8. This section was used to assess the effects of time constraints on the accuracy shown in recalling the target levels. In previous sections, the subject was free to begin a contraction at any time after the announcement of the colour. In this section, the colour was announced and then the subject had to observe a delay which randomly varied from one to ten seconds. At the end of the specified delay he was told to tense up immediately. The recall procedure was, in all other respects, the same as that outlined in Section 4.

Results

The polygraph records were scored in the way described in Experiment 3. Figures 9 and 10 show the accuracy of performance achieved at various stages during training. The error was computed by taking the difference (in EMG units) between the level produced and the target level; no account was taken of the direction of error. All five subjects were able to attain criterion accuracy in the various sections and to complete the training programme.

Analyses of variance were used to compare the recall accuracy shown in Section 2 and that produced after training in Section 3. Figure 9 shows that a significant improvement was achieved in the appropriateness of the activity levels which were produced ($F = 14.10$; df $= 2,8$; $p < 0.01$). A corresponding reduction in error is shown in Fig. 10; again this was found to be significant ($F = 21.66$; df $= 1,4$; $p < 0.01$). In Section 4, subjects were asked to recall the targets that they had learned in Section 3, but this time they had to switch from one target to another. A loss in accuracy was observed, which was not surprising in view of the delay after training and the extra demands made. The loss in accuracy did not reach significance ($p > 0.05$) when the levels produced, or the errors incurred, were compared. The effects of training subjects to switch from one target to another whilst producing each accurately can be assessed by comparing the performances produced in Sections 4 and 6. Figure 9 shows that an improvement in recall accuracy was achieved for the Black and White targets. An analysis of variance showed that the improvement in over-all accuracy was significant ($F = 5.14$; df $= 2,8$; $p < 0.05$). However, the corresponding decrease in error failed to reach significance (p > 0.05). Sections 6 and 8 differed only with respect to the time constraints imposed in the latter; this did not impair performance. Indeed, when subjects altered their performance, they did so in the direction of achieving greater accuracy; over-all, these changes did not reach significance (p > 0.05). A reduction in the time taken to recapture criterion performance is also evidence of learning. Table I compares the number of attempts which were needed before criterion accuracy was achieved in Sections 5 and 7. Apart from Sp 4, all subjects needed fewer attempts in order to regain the accuracy that they had achieved in Section 5.

TABLE I

The number of attempts produced before criterion performance was achieved in Sections 5 and 7

Section	Sp 1	Sp 2	Sp 3	Sp 4	Sp 5
5	124	46	37	17	28
7	40	45	2	43	6

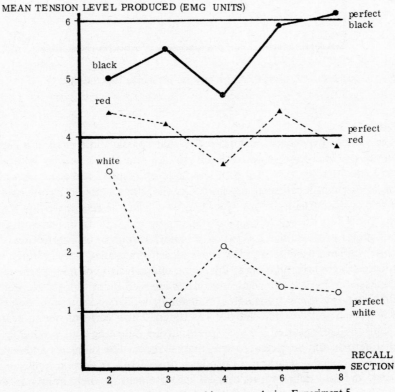

Fig. 9. The recall accuracy achieved by the spastic subject group during Experiment 5.

89

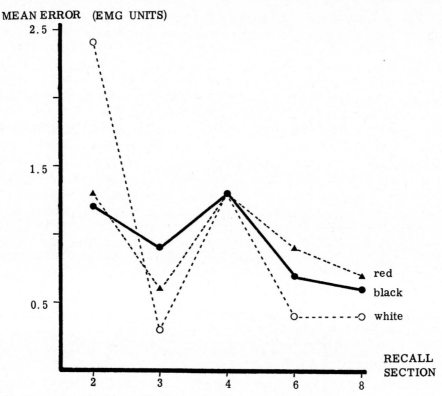

Fig. 10. The recall accuracy achieved by the spastic subject during Experiment 5.

Discussion

The present experiment demonstrates that spastic individuals are capable of learning to produce representative levels of fore-arm flexor activity with stringent accuracy when they are provided with knowledge of results. The accuracy which they showed in the final recall sections was better than that achieved in previous studies by neurologically normal persons when they were asked to repeat tension levels. The training procedure therefore enabled the spastic individuals to learn to construct accurate motor programmes and to control relevant sources of interference. At first, the spastic subjects overshot the low levels of neuromuscular activity which were set and underestimated the high ones, this being characteristic of their performance on previous tasks. However, knowledge of results enabled them to learn to produce the low and high target levels accurately. Immediately following Section 8, each subject's ability to scale neuromuscular activity was tested. Their performance indicated that these subjects had acquired a lower threshold for detecting and producing neuro-muscular activity and an increased sensitivity to error. The subjects had been able to use their experience of learning to produce three levels of fore-arm flexor activity accurately and had achieved an over-all improvement in their ability to evaluate and regulate neuromuscular activity. Although the knowledge of results that was

90

given was crude, in the sense that it told the subject only whether his attempt was too high or too low, it did provide him with all the information he needed to learn to control muscular activity with the stringent accuracy which was demanded.

The timing constraints imposed in Section 8 referred only to the initiation of a response and not to its completion. The results indicate that the spastic individual is not forced into inaccuracy when he is no longer free to choose when a contraction is begun. No assessment was made of whether spastic persons are able to learn to programme a contraction so that a particular level of activity is achieved at a specific moment in time. If they are unable to do so, this will restrict the temporal patterns of muscular activity which they can produce and the types and speeds of movement that they are able to use.

In the case of the fore-arm flexor muscle group, spastic individuals demonstrated that they do have a potential for achieving better motor control. It is always possible that this muscle group is in some way atypical and that a similar improvement would not have been achieved with other groups. The next experiment therefore investigated whether spastic subjects are also able to control the biceps muscle accurately. In addition, it investigated whether they are capable of learning to control more complex patterns of neuromuscular activity.

Experiment 6: Training spastic individuals to control the activity of both the fore-arm flexor and biceps muscles accurately

Normal movements typically involve the contraction of a large number of muscles. To perform these accurately, an individual must be capable of regulating and evaluating the activity of constituent muscle groups precisely and of preserving this control when other contractions are simultaneously present. The present experiment was designed to investigate whether spastic individuals are capable of learning to produce specified patterns of sequential and simultaneous activity in the biceps and fore-arm flexor muscle groups. Knowledge of results was provided to help them to learn to produce these accurately. These tasks represent an extension of the cognitive demands made upon the spastic subject, for he must learn to evaluate and regulate activity in two muscle groups and he must learn to control simultaneous contractions. It is unlikely that the spastic individual will be able to achieve a pattern of simultaneous activity simply by running the two motor programmes which were successful in producing the relevant contractions in isolation. It is known that the voluntary contraction of the biceps muscle often creates fore-arm flexor activity in the spastic neuromusculature and *vice versa*. The spastic individual must therefore learn to take account of induced activity, otherwise he will overshoot the activity levels which are required. In some instances, spastic individuals may have to find methods of inhibiting induced activity before they are able to achieve the patterns of neuromuscular activity specified.

Procedure

The general procedure closely followed that adopted in Experiment 5. Surface electrodes were attached in order to record from the biceps and fore-arm flexor muscles, and subjects were helped to identify these groups. The sensitivity of the

91

apparatus was adjusted until the reliable maximum contraction that a subject was able to produce in both of the muscle groups occupied seven EMG units of the recording paper. The target levels of neuromuscular activity consisted of a high and a low level of activity in the fore-arm flexor and biceps muscles. Extreme levels were chosen because these had proved the most difficult for a subject to learn to control in the previous experiment. The following colour code was adopted:—

Muscle	EMG units	Colour
Fore-arm flexors	6	Black (B)
	1	White (W)
Biceps	5	Brown (BR)
	2	Yellow (Y)

SECTION 1. In this section, subjects were taught to produce all four specified levels of neuromuscular activity accurately. The subject was given a copy of Fig. 11 and the experimenter explained that the Brown and Black targets represented high levels of muscular activity whilst the White and Yellow targets involved low levels. The order in which the colours were trained was randomised, the only constraint being that muscle groups were alternated. The definition of a correct performance and the form of knowledge of results that was used were the same as those adopted in Experiment 5. Each target was separately trained. The subject made repeated attempts to produce a target and was given feedback as to his accuracy; this was continued until he produced three successive correct responses. Immediate recall was tested by asking him to produce five examples of the learned target; no feedback was given at this point. When all four targets had been learned and immediate recall tested, the next section followed immediately.

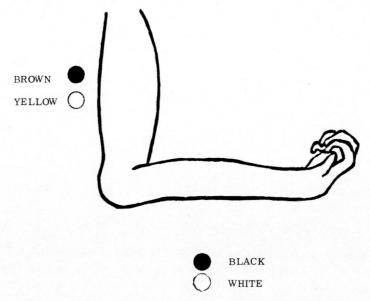

Fig. 11. The target guide provided for subjects in Experiment 6.

SECTION 2. This section tested the subject's ability to recall the four targets. The subject completed five trials; in each of these he was aksed to produce all four targets in randomised order. No feedback was given; a short rest followed before the next section was begun.

SECTION 3. In this section, subjects were trained to switch from one target to another, producing each of them accurately. Lists were prepared that consisted of blocks, each of which contained all four colours in randomised order. The subject worked through a list and was given knowledge of results about the accuracy of each attempt. This continued until the subject managed to produce two successive blocks correctly, *i.e.,* eight successive accurate target levels. The next section followed immediately.

SECTION 4. This was a repeat of Section 2.

SECTION 5. This section tested the subject's ability to produce specified levels of simultaneous activity in the biceps and fore-arm flexor muscle groups. Subjects were given any clarification that was necessary as to the meaning of the word 'simultaneous'. The experimenter stressed that a subject was free to take as long as he wished adjusting muscular activity; when he felt that the required combination was present, the subject said 'now'. The combinations which were tested were as follows:

B/Y   = high fore-arm flexor—low biceps activity
B/BR = high fore-arm flexor—high biceps activity
W/Y = low fore-arm flexor—low biceps activity
W/BR = low fore-arm flexor—high biceps activity

The subject made five successive attempts at producing a particular pattern of simultaneous activity; he was given no feedback as to his accuracy. The order in which the targets were demanded was randomised.

SECTION 6. This section was designed to teach the subject to produce all four patterns of simultaneous activity correctly. A particular combination was taken and the subject trained to produce it accurately; his immediate recall of this was then tested. The order in which the four combinations were tested was randomised. When a combination was specified and when feedback was given, the fore-arm flexor group was always mentioned first. Knowledge of results would therefore be given as follows: Black, high; Brown, low. The subject made repeated attempts at a particular combination until he produced three successive correct responses. Immediate recall was tested by asking him to produce five examples of the trained response; no feedback was given at this point.

Results

The polygraph records were scored in the way described in Experiment 3. Figures 12 and 13 show the accuracy of performance achieved at various stages during training. All five subjects were able to attain criterion accuracy in the various sections and to complete the training programme.

Poorer recall accuracy was observed in Section 2 than in Section 1. This is not surprising because more time had elapsed since training and targets were now being demanded in a randomised order. An analysis of variance was used to compare the mean levels of integrated activity that were produced in the two sections; these were not found to differ significantly ($p > 0.05$). A second analysis of variance compared the errors produced; the difference between the two sections just failed to reach significance ($F = 7.63$; df $= 1,4$; $p = 0.051$). During Section 3, subjects were trained to switch from one target to another, producing each of them accurately. This experience brought about a marked improvement in their recall accuracy. An analysis of variance showed a significant improvement in the accuracy of the attempts made during Section 4 ($F = 4.56$; df $= 3,12$; $p < 0.05$). A corresponding reduction in error was found ($F = 13.13$; df $= 1,4$; $p < 0.05$) when the performances in Sections 2 and 4 were compared.

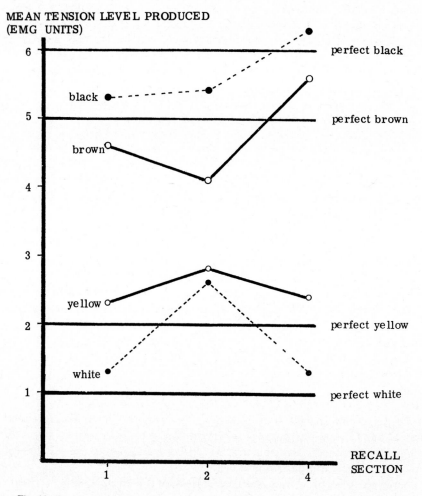

Fig. 12. The recall accuracy achieved by the spastic subject group during Experiment 6.

In order to assess the effects of training on the spastic subjects' ability to produce simultaneous patterns of activity, a single index of their accuracy had to be developed. This was achieved by summating the errors shown in producing the individual targets. Table II compares the errors produced by the spastic subjects in Sections 5 and 6.

An analysis of variance indicated that a significant improvement in the subjects' ability to produce simultaneous levels of neuromuscular activity followed the training given in Section 6 (F = 26.84; df = 1,4; p < 0.01).

TABLE II
The mean summated error scores (EMG units) produced in Sections 5 and 6

| | Target combinations | | | |
	Black / Yellow	Black / Brown	White / Yellow	White / Brown
Section 5	4.62	5.68	2.74	5.06
Section 6	1.26	1.16	0.55	1.13

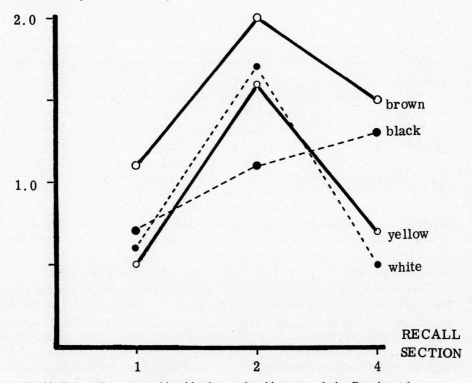

Fig. 13. The recall accuracy achieved by the spastic subject group during Experiment 6.

95

A description of the levels of activity present in the fore-arm flexor and biceps muscles during Section 3, when subjects were concentrating on producing individual targets, was undertaken. Subjects were able to switch from one muscle group to another accurately, and it was therefore assumed that the simultaneous activity which was observed in the irrelevant group was induced by the prime contraction. For each subject, the levels of biceps and fore-arm flexor activity present for every attempt at a target were noted. The pairs of data obtained when fore-arm flexor targets were being aimed for were analysed to find the linear or exponential equation which best fitted the relationship observed between fore-arm flexor activity and induced biceps activity. This equation was used to compute the levels of biceps activity which were induced when the White and Black targets were being produced. A similar computation was followed to find the levels of fore-arm flexor activity induced by the Brown and Yellow targets. The data for each of the spastic individuals are given in Table III.

TABLE III

The levels of muscular activity (EMG units) induced by the flexor and biceps targets during Section 3

	Induced biceps activity (EMG units)		Induced fore-arm flexor activity (EMG units)	
	Black	White	Brown	Yellow
Sp 1	3.5	0.3	5.6	4.8
Sp 2	3.2	0.2	5.0	1.8
Sp 3	2.0	0.0	3.6	1.8
Sp 4	3.3	0.3	3.7	0.5
Sp 5	6.8	0.2	5.5	3.8

Table III indicates that as a higher level of activity was produced in a muscle, the level of activity induced in the other also rose. In many instances, the levels of induced activity were too high for the required patterns of simultaneous activity to be produced. This suggests that, in these cases, subjects had to learn to suppress induced activity before they were able to reach criterion accuracy in Section 6. Only Sp 3 displayed a level of induced biceps activity which was low enough for him to produce the Black/Yellow combination without first suppressing some biceps activity. Indeed, Sp 5 showed a level of induced biceps activity which would have precluded his attaining the Black/Brown combination. In order to achieve the White/Brown targets, all subjects had to reduce the level of fore-arm flexor activity that was induced. Only Sp 4 might be expected to produce the White and Yellow targets simultaneously without first suppressing some induced flexor activity.

In an attempt to represent the performance of subjects during Section 6, when they were attempting to produce accurate patterns of simultaneous activity, 'form curves' were produced. The technique for doing so has been described elsewhere (Harrison and Connolly 1971). In broad terms, the attempts at producing a particular combination were partitioned into six sequential segments which contained, as far as possible, an equal number of attempts. The mean levels of biceps and fore-arm flexor activity observed during a segment were computed. Figure 14 shows the changes in

96

muscular activity which occurred as subjects learned to produce the prescribed combination more accurately. The form curves shown may be an imperfect representation of individual performances because the data for the group have been pooled. However, the raw data for individual subjects appeared to be in the broad agreement with the changes shown in Fig. 14. As Section 6 progressed, subjects gradually pared induced activity until it was appropriate to the target combination. Some subjects at first expressed doubt as to whether they would be able to reduce excess activity but with persistence they were able to do so. The systematic improvement shown would support the view that they were intelligently using the knowledge of results which they were given and that success did not come simply by chance.

Subject Sp 4 found it difficult to produce certain patterns of simultaneous activity because of the effects of surgery which had been directed at limiting elbow movement. The resulting fore-arm posture meant that wrist flexion created elbow flexion. This subject therefore had great difficulty in producing the Black/Yellow combination accurately.

The subjects' ability to recall individual targets was most accurate during Section 1. Table IV compares the precision which would have been expected if they managed to retain this accuracy when set the task of producing simultaneous contractions with that actually observed in Section 6.

Table IV indicates that the subjects actually produced certain targets *more* accurately, when these were demanded in combination, than might have been predicted from their Section 1 performance. Despite the increased demands made of the subjects, the combinations involving a high level of biceps activity were more accurately produced in Section 6. This could be due to a simple practice effect, but it is more likely that uncontrolled movements of the other joint were an important source of error when subjects were attempting to produce individual targets in Section 1. The feedback which was given in Section 6 enabled the subjects to define the functional link between fore-arm flexor and biceps activity. With this information, they were able to take account of induced activity when programming targets and so they produced them more accurately.

TABLE IV

A comparison between the summated error scores (EMG units) observed in Section 6 and those predicted from Section 1 performance (Experiment 6)

	Black/Brown	Black/Yellow	White/Brown	White/Yellow
Section 1	1.8	1.2	1.7	1.1
Section 6	1.2	1.3	0.6	1.2

Discussion

A limb movement may be described as a series of muscular contractions each of a specific strength which occur in a particular temporal sequence. Figure 15 represents a movement which consists of activity in the biceps and fore-arm flexor muscles. Experiments 5 and 6 investigated whether spastic individuals can be taught to produce component contractions accurately. The first study showed that they can learn to produce a wide range of neuromuscular activity levels accurately. The second experiment showed that spastic persons can be taught to programme sequential and

97

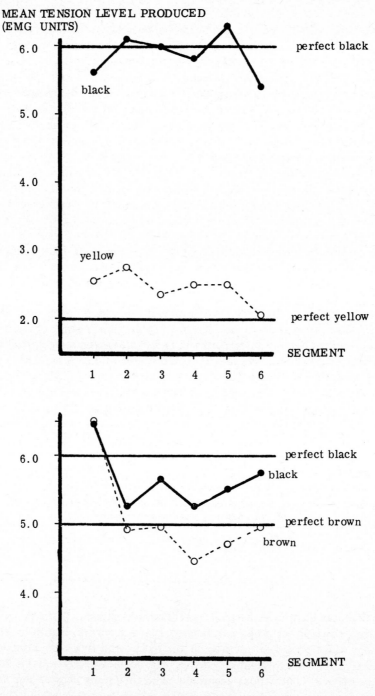

Fig. 14 (*and see facing page*). 'Form curves' showing the development of accuracy in producing simultaneous levels of activity in the fore-arm flexor and biceps muscle groups (Experiment 6).

MEAN TENSION LEVEL PRODUCED
(EMG UNITS)

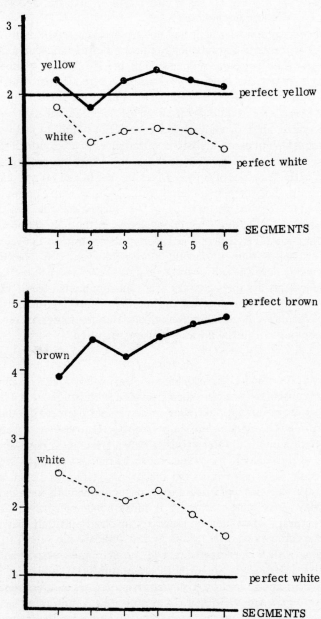

simultaneous activity in two muscle groups with an accuracy comparable to that to be expected from neurologically normal subjects. Taken together, these experiments demonstrate that spastic individuals are capable of producing the patterns of muscular activity specified at stages Y and Z and of making the switch from one muscle group to another demanded at X.

A necessary requirement which has not so far been established is that spastic persons have a potential for producing patterns of neuromuscular activity which conform to a specified temporal sequence. Further studies are planned which will investigate whether they can learn to programme contractions so that the muscular activity builds up at a specified rate, reaches its peak at the correct time and declines at a stipulated speed. A system other than verbal feedback will be required to train subjects to produce appropriately timed contractions and to achieve particular temporal relationships between activity in different muscle groups. Tracking is one method which might be used; this provides the subject simultaneously with a representation of the sequence of activity which he should aim for and that which he is actually producing. This system therefore provides him with continuous feedback about the accuracy of his performance. The success of the last two training experiments suggests that knowledge of results is, in the long term, a more useful form of feedback for the spastic subject, for it allows him to concentrate fully on constructing an appropriate movement programme and on detecting accurate inherent movement cues. The spastic individual may learn to track more precisely but may be unable to replicate this accuracy when the augmented feedback is removed. The experiments which are planned use the paradigm of asking the spastic individual to produce a particular sequence of muscular activity and afterwards showing how his performance compares with the pattern that was required.

SUMMARY

The present experiments demonstrate that spastic individuals do have a potential for better neuromuscular control. When provided with augmented feedback, they learned to relax more quickly and showed some improvement in their ability to maintain specific levels of neuromuscular activity. Knowledge of results enabled spastic subjects to achieve normal precision when producing high, low and intermediate levels of muscular activity. They also learned to produce sequential and simultaneous patterns of activity in the biceps and fore-arm flexor muscles with stringent accuracy. Before it can be said that spastic individuals have the potential to perform everyday tasks more normally, it must be demonstrated that they can maintain this accuracy when more muscles are involved and that they can learn to meet temporal specifications. The results to date indicate the value of providing the spastic individual with a clear assessment of the neuromuscular activity that he is producing. First, it provides him with the opportunity of achieving a functional definition of his neuromusculature and of identifying sources of interference. Secondly, it permits him to experiment with ways of suppressing unwanted activity and to evaluate different movement programmes. The challenge for the future is to design training programmes which will enable spastic individuals to realise their full potential for neuromuscular control.

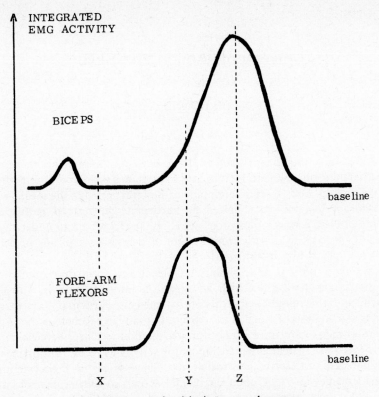

Fig. 15. Pattern of activity in two muscle groups.

Acknowledgements

Iam grateful to the Spastics Society for the provision of the equipment used in these studies, and also to my subjects for their hard work.
I would also like to thank Keven Connolly for his guidance and criticism.

REFERENCES

Harrison, A. (1973) 'Studies of neuromuscular control in spastic persons.' Unpublished Ph.D. thesis, Sheffield University.
—— Connolly, K. (1971) 'The conscious control of fine levels of neuromuscular firing in spastic and normal subjects.' *Developmental Medicine and Child Neurology,* **13,** 762.
Netsell, R., Cleeland, C. S. (1973) 'Modification of lip hypertonia in dysarthria using EMG feedback.' *Journal of Speech and Hearing Disorders,* **38,** 131.
Phillips, C. G. (1969) 'Motor apparatus of the baboon's hand.' *Proceedings of the Royal Society, Series B,* **173,** 141.

CHAPTER EIGHT

Movement, Action and Skill

KEVIN CONNOLLY

The notion of development is protean, for as each of us approaches the concept it assumes different forms. Sometimes it is used to connote a process and sometimes the product of a process. Growth and development, however, provide the means whereby a child achieves the necessary power to participate in human culture. Some appreciation of these very complex processes is essential if we are to understand how the human being goes so quickly from a state of helplessness to one of achieving mastery over much of his environment.

Motor activity itself is of enormous biological and social importance since it provides the principal ways in which an organism interacts with its surrounding environment and also operates upon its environment in particular ways to achieve desired ends. An analysis of much of the current thinking in psychology shows that we fail to consider mental activities in their proper relation to motor behaviour. Sperry (1952) puts this well: 'Instead of regarding motor activity as being subsidiary, that is, something to carry out, serve, and satisfy the demands of the higher centres, we reverse this tendency and look upon the mental activity as only a means to an end, where the end is a better regulation of the overt response. Cerebration, essentially, serves to bring into motor behavior additional refinement, increased direction toward distant future goals, and greater over-all adaptiveness and survival value. The evolutionary increase in man's capacity for perception, feeling, ideation, imagination and the like, may be regarded not so much as an end in itself but as something that has enabled us to behave, to act, more wisely and efficiently'.

Turning an accepted way of looking at the world on its head as Sperry does is both revealing and illuminating.

The literature on the development of skills in infancy and childhood is sparse, but the situation is much worse with regard to theories of action and of skill development. For the most part the literature on motor development is concerned with the achievement of norms rather than with a careful and precise description of behaviour. My concern is primarily with the development of skills and I propose to address myself to the question of how we should consider the relationship of movement to skill and the acquisition of skill in infancy.

Movements are of biological significance to the organism in that they make up acts which solve motor problems. Such problems arise usually in the external environment (Bernstein 1967). The distinction between actions and movements is an important one which is often not fully appreciated. When we speak of skills—walking, crawling, grasping, *etc.*—we refer to the organisation of certain movements into a purposeful plan which is executed with economy. An essential attribute of skill lies in the ability to achieve a goal, because skilled activity is *purposeful*. Another feature of behaviour which we describe as skilled is its flexibility and this too is an ubiquitous property. In various skills, for example, walking over uneven ground, jumping over obstacles or swimming through waves, the individual is engaged in overcoming independent forces. This draws a distinction between meaningful actions and a range of independent movements which are not concerned with overcoming external forces. Overcoming these external forces is a prerequisite for the solution of motor problems and since they are not forseeable they cannot be overcome in any stereotyped way.

In order to draw out further the relationship between movements, actions and skills, let us consider an example. Imagine writing the initial letter of your name, first with a pencil held in your preferred hand and writing on a sheet of paper, and then with a pencil tied to the end of a broom handle which would require the use of two hands to write on a vertical surface. Both of these tasks we can accomplish and the skill in question is writing. But notice that quite different sets of muscles are involved; we arrive at the same end product via quite different routes. If we think of the child learning to write we can see that this involves not only learning a sequence of appropriate postures and movements, but also some higher level description in which the child must learn about writing in terms of a temporal and spatial sequence of strokes. With writing then we may suppose that the brain accumulates high-level routines in terms of variously directed motions on the basis of relative position without any specific reference to absolute position (Arbib 1972). Insofar as a high-level programme is available, it is possible to execute fairly skilled movements even though they have not been performed previously.

Skilled activity may be thought of as a programme of action directed towards the attainment of some goal (Connolly 1973). If we think of skills as programmes of events purposefully organised, then basic questions concern the units making up the programme and how these units are organised. Although motor problems require movements for their solution, the units in an action programme are not themselves movements. I have argued elsewhere (Connolly 1970) that action programmes are made up of a serially-ordered set of constituent sub-routines. A sub-routine is an act, the performance of which is a necessary, but not sufficient, condition for the execution of some more complex, hierarchically-organised sequence of sub-routines of which it is a member (Elliott and Connolly 1974). A whole sequence of correctly organised actions constitutes what is generally thought of as a skill, *e.g.* walking, singing, playing the piano or using a tool such as a screwdriver. The sub-routine then gains its significance as an act from the context in which it occurs. Thus skill is modular, and the distinction between problem-solving and skilled performance might be seen as the distinction between the organisation and execution of sub-routines (Elliott and Connolly 1974). Again the relationship between movement and action presents itself. Nerve impulses and muscle contractions, though necessary for action and skilled motor behaviour are better seen as accompaniments of action rather than characteristics of it. The defining characteristic of an act is intentionality, but this is not a defining characteristic of muscle fibres. It is reasonable to say, 'I intend to turn the page of this manuscript'. This is something which I choose to do, but I do not choose to transmit nerve impulses or contract a particular sub-set of extrafusal and

103

intrafusal muscle fibres.*

As I have argued in the example above of writing the initial letter of my name, there is no necessary identity between a particular constellation of muscle contractions brought into play in the performance of an act and the act itself. An act such as writing the letter 'C', or a skill such as walking, is more than the sum of its parts because it has consequences. Changes are brought about in the environment as a consequence of the movements which make up the action. Given that there is no identity between movements and actions (because the latter can be achieved by a variety of means (for example, writing the letter 'C'), how can the vast array of movement patterns which an individual might employ be stored in the brain? The answer, of course, is that they are not, no more than all the possible sentences which can be constructed in the English language are stored in the brain. Language is generative; a minimum set of transformation rules serve to produce a vast array of utterances, and similarly, a large stock of skilled action patterns may be generated in achieving a wide variety of goals. The analogy with linguistics is interesting and illuminating. On the basis of Chomsky's (1965) theory the individual is presumed to have at his disposal an abstract system which is referred to as the 'deep structure', this set of organising principles allows him to generate and to understand an indefinite but very large set of sentences called the 'surface structure'. Although the deep structure determines the surface structure, it is not manifest in it. This position is similar to that advanced by Bernstein (1967) in discussing what he calls the 'motor-image', '... the higher engram of a given topological class, is already structurally extremely far removed (and because of this also probably localizationally very distant) from any resemblance whatever to the joint-muscle schemata; it is extremely geometrical, representing a very abstract motor image of space'.

Bernstein's view is that the central substrate or engram for a pattern of movements is some representation of the environment.

Given that voluntary movements take place, the question is *how*. Coupled with this, we have a further theoretical problem in understanding how voluntary action and skill develop in infancy and childhood. Bartlett (1958) wrote of the skilled operator as having 'all the time in the world to do what he wants'. The concern here with timing is not with the absolute speed at which any component in a skilled action can be performed but with regulating the flow of behaviour from component to component: '... nowhere in the whole series is there any appearance of hurry and nowhere unnecessarily prolonged delay ...' (Bartlett 1958). The secret of the smooth action which so characterises the highly skilled performer involves anticipation and fitting acts into a previously determined serial programme. This leads to problems of control. One of the crucial features involved in the regulation of intentional voluntary action concerns the opportunity to compare what was intended with the outcome, so that any discrepancy may be turned into a correction signal, and the behaviour then modified as necessary.

A number of models have been described which provide the basic logic of a control system. An early approach to these problems is reflected in the pioneering

*Exceptions to this general statement may come to light following the work of Hefferline (1958), Basmajian (1963) and Harrison and Connolly (1971). See Harrison's chapters in this volume.

104

work of von Holst and Mittelstaedt (1950, *and* von Holst 1954) who developed the concept of reafference. This approach was subsequently modified and elaborated upon by Hein and Held (1962). For a review of these see Connolly (1969). A similar, though in some ways more developed model has been offered by Bernstein (1967). Bernstein argues that any system which is self-regulating must incorporate the following elements as minimum requirements:

(1) *effector* (motor) activity, which is regulated along the given parameter;
(2) *a control element,* which conveys to the system in one way or another the required value of the parameter which is to be regulated;
(3) *a receptor,* which perceives the factual course of the value of the parameter and signals it by some means to
(4) *a comparator device,* which perceives the discrepancy between the factual and required values with its magnitude and sign;
(5) *an apparatus,* which encodes the data provided by the comparator device into correlation impulses which are transmitted by feedback linkages to
(6) *a regulator,* which controls the function of the effector along a given parameter.

The required value of the parameter to be regulated is known as the *sollwert* (Sw), the factual course of the parameter is known as the *istwert* (Iw) and any discrepancy perceived by the comparator device is known as the *deltawert* (Δw). The model is presents itself. Nerve impulses and muscle contractions, though necessary for action and skilled motor behaviour, are better seen as accompaniments of action rather than from the realised action (istwert, Iw), these being used to generate the crucial discrepancy (deltawert, Δw) which is then translated into the necessary correction signal. The central and most problematic feature of all of this is the control element, the programmes which signal the intended sollwert.

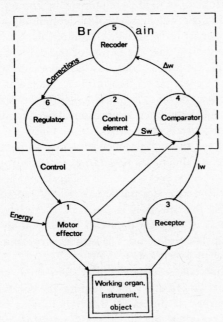

Fig. 1. Bernstein's model of a control system capable of voluntary action directed towards objects or states of the environment (modified after Bruner 1970).

105

The major part of understanding how voluntary movement takes place, *i.e.* understanding how action patterns are realised, lies with our appreciation of this control element and with the concept of feed-forward. Feed-forward has been defined as, 'A method of control in which disturbances affecting output variables are anticipated and compensating fluctuations of the input variables are generated' (Meetham 1969). In other words, it has to do with using a model to predict what is about to happen, so that the outcome of a series of movements can be computed before the outcome materialises. Movement is thus transformed into action by some form of imaging process which is presumed to occur in the motor cortex. Pribram (1971) has called this an 'image-of-achievement'. Such an image-of-achievement contains all input and outcome information for the next step in the realisation of the action pattern.

The essential feature of all this is that properties of the environment—and not configurations of muscles and joints—become cortically encoded. Bernstein's (1967) observations, based upon his careful description of changes in walking as a function of age, suggest that constancy can be achieved in action regardless of particular movements or the amount of contraction in a particular muscle group. He argued that the topological properties of space are represented in the motor cortex. This turned out to be wrong, as Evarts (1967) has demonstrated experimentally. Instead, the forces exciting muscle receptors are represented cortically. Action is thus possible because movements become attuned to the field of external forces. Pribram (1971) has suggested that this cortical representation can be thought of as a mirror-image of the field of external forces. An interesting feature of Pribram's formulation is that action and consequence are inseparable not only conceptually but also neuro-physiologically.

Let me now return to the problem of skill development in infancy. To use the analogy with language, once again the problem is one of understanding how the child gets from his very limited experience with the surface structure (his extremely limited repertoire of actions) to one of understanding the nature of the deep structure. How does he come to perform actions by various routes, where does my constancy in writing the letter 'C' in various ways come from? Sub-routines, viewed as components of action, have two sources of origin; they may be pre-adapted in the genome or they may be individuated from the undifferentiated expression of an intention through some motor action which is appropriate in a gross sense. Once an action plan emerges, it can be shaped and refined through practice. Practice, as Bernstein (1967) argued, does not consist in repeating the *means of solution* of a motor problem but repeating the *process of solving,* by techniques which are changed and perfected from repetition to repetition. Thus '... practice is a particular type of repetition without repetition and motor training, if this position is ignored, is merely mechanical repetition by rote ...'. The process of practice then can be seen as the search for optimal motor solutions to appropriate problems. The central programme itself thus changes, not merely the means of its execution.

Over the course of development, each encounter the child has with his surrounding environment presents conditions which require the solution of motor problems. In some manner which we do not as yet understand, this results in the development within the nervous system of reliable and accurate objective representations of the external world. Initial learning is based upon a substantial amount of pre-adaptation which reflects species-typic genetic instructions and the whole process of primate evolution. Unlike *Topsy,* we, that is the species, did not simply grow, but were shaped and designed by environmental pressures and genetic adaptations over long periods. During development, initial acts and patterns of action become constituents for new patterns directed at goals which are more remote and often far more complex. A fundamental problem is thus concerned with initial plans, or, as Bruner (1973) puts it, with the 'initial arousal of intention' by an appropriate object. How, and by what physiological means, the image of an envisioned movement functions as a guiding principle of the structure of an act, we do not know at present.

That intention exists in the infant is not in question. Its existence has, for example, been demonstrated by Bower *et al.* (1970), and Bruner (1973) has listed several measurable attributes: (1) anticipation of outcome of an act; (2) selection of appropriate means to achieve the end state; (3) sustained direction of behaviour during deployment of means; (4) a stop order defined by a given end state; (5) substitution rules whereby alternative means can be deployed for the correction of deviations. By virtue of these capacities, Bruner argues that the infant's behaviour which initially occurs 'reflexively' and 'instinctually' is converted into intentional action when the infant has the opportunity to obtain knowledge of results. The consequences of the infant's behaviour become important factors in refining actions. On the basis of a series of very elegant and insightful observations, Bruner puts the case as follows (Bruner and Koslowski 1972, Bruner 1973).

'Initial arousal is often followed by a loosely ordered sequence of constituent acts that will later occur in an appropriate serial order to achieve the end state towards which intention appears to be steering. Meanwhile, during this clumsy athetoid phase, the consummatory response will continue, and even the wrongly-orchestrated constituent acts can be shown to have an appropriate adjustment with respect to the goal. The development of visually-guided reaching is typical of this pattern. An appropriate free-standing object, of appropriate size and texture and at an appropriate distance, first produces prolonged looking and, very shortly after, there is action of the mouth and tongue and jaws—the area to which a captured object will be transported once effective, visually-guided reaching develops. If the infant persists, one can then observe antigravitational activity of arms and shoulders, clenching of fists in a "grab" pattern, movement of arms, ballistic flinging of clenched fists, etc.'.

Given that the constituent components of action are present, they may be organised into various serial arrays. The practice of an action in the presence of an appropriate 'releasing stimulus' gives rise to feed-back (from effectors), thus allowing for the establishment of co-ordination between feed-forward signals and peripheral feed-back. Eventually the act is successfully executed and an object is grasped and carried to the mouth. The process of solution of this motor problem can then be practised and refined, and reinforcement from knowledge of results can further shape the act.

Complex motor behaviour may be viewed as the building up of sub-structures each of which deals with a limited aspect of the problem. If we choose to think of motor acts in this way, then it follows that an important task is to isolate the sub-structures of motor behaviour and investigate ways in which they are combined to produce co-ordinated action patterns. Arbib (1972) has outlined a basic hierarchical model (Fig. 2). Here an action is dependent upon a gross command which is tuned primarily by measurements of local conditions and also by high-level commands being sent to adjacent levels. These commands need only be, to use Greene's (1972) vivid terminology, 'in the right ball-park'. Given that the gross command is sufficiently close to the desired trajectory, then the tuning inputs can refine and modulate the output. An example provided by Arbib (1972) concerns the idea of a postural frame within which movements take place: 'Lower level feedback via spinal reflexes can serve to keep an animal from falling over despite changing support conditions. Commands to move need not carry information about what will happen to the center of gravity if a certain leg is lifted—the postural "tuning inputs" will cause the whole body (if necessary) to move so as to provide proper support. Parallel command paths can then impose refinements (such as the finger movements involved in playing the piano) upon the gross trajectory with feedback stabilisation'.

I have argued that in understanding motor skill and how it develops it is necessary for us to appreciate the proper relationship between action and movement. There is no *identity* between action and movement. A given set of muscle contractions does not in itself define a skill because a skill is more than the sum of its constituent parts. The co-ordination of movements into purposeful goal-orientated programmes of action involves the intention to achieve a goal and the presence of a control system which can shape and refine both the behaviour and the driving programme.

During the course of development, various changes of constraint will operate differentially on the realisation of motor behaviour. Broadly, these constraints could be distinguished as hardware and software changes (Connolly 1970, 1973). Maturational changes within the nervous system and biomechanical changes in the limbs and body as a whole will affect the expression of skill. Along with these changes there will be other changes of a cognitive kind, having to do with components of action (the sub-routines referred to earlier). The assembly of the basic building blocks of skill (sub-routines), and the learning of transformation rules by which the units are

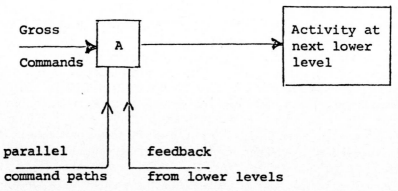

Fig. 2. Basic hierarchical model illustrating means of providing tuning inputs for movements triggered by gross commands (from Arbib 1972).

108

governed and mobilised in executing action programmes, lies at the heart of our understanding of the growth of skill.

At the beginning of this paper I referred to the paucity of theory with respect to skill development. The lack of any adequate theoretical formulation to guide empirical work is significant not only for the advancement of biological and psychological science, but also for a better understanding of the problems of the handicapped. For the most part, science advances significantly when its practitioners ask better, more pertinent, more powerful questions. How we formulate questions in applied fields is no less significant. Pribram *et al.* (1955) published a report of studies in which they investigated some effects of ablating the motor cortex in monkeys. Following this procedure the animals were observed to be clumsy in performing the skilled sequences of action involved in opening latches and boxes. However, when these animals were filmed climbing on the mesh sides of their cages or grooming, it became apparent that they were able to perform exactly those finger and hand movements required for opening the latches without any undue difficulty. Thus, only some acts and achievements were difficult, and the difficulty which the animals experienced had little to do with specific movements. Our understanding of how systems function is by no means irrelevant to developing better medical and social care, and to devising techniques of therapy and training with which to help the handicapped and the crippled to achieve competence and control over their environment.

Acknowledgements

I am grateful to Margaret Martlew for discussing with me the analogies between language and skill. The ideas put forward in this paper developed over the course of a research programme supported by the Spastics Society, London.

Fig. 2 was taken from *The Metaphorical Brain* by M. A. Arbib, 1972, and was reproduced by kind permission of John Wiley and Sons Ltd.

REFERENCES

Arbib, M. A. (1972) *The Metaphorical Brain. An Introduction to Cybernetics as Artificial Intelligence and Brain Theory.* London/New York: Wiley.

Bartlett, F. C. (1958) *Thinking: An Experimental and Social Study.* London: Allen and Unwin.

Basmajian, J. V. (1963) 'Control and training of individual motor units.' *Science,* **141,** 440.

Bernstein, N. (1967) *The Co-ordination and Regulation of Movements.* Oxford/New York: Pergamon Press.

Bower, T. G. R., Broughton, J. M., Moore, M. K. (1970) 'Demonstration of intention in the reaching behaviour of neonate humans.' *Nature,* **228,** 679.

Bruner, J. S. (1970) 'The growth and structure of skill.' *In* Connolly, K. J. (Ed.) *Mechanisms of Motor Skill Development.* London/New York: Academic Press.

—— (1973) Organisation of early skilled action.' *Child Development,* **44,** 1.

—— Koslowski, B. (1972) 'Visually preadapted constituents of manipulatory action.' *Perception,* **1,** 3.

Chomsky, N. (1965) *Aspects of the Theory of Syntax.* Cambridge, Mass.: M.I.T. Press.

Connolly, K. (1969) 'Sensory-motor co-ordination: mechanisms and plans.' *In* Wolff, P., Mac Keith, R. (Eds.) *Planning for Better Learning.* Clinics in Developmental Medicine, no. 33. London: Spastics International Medical Publications with Heinemann Medical.

—— (1970) 'Skill development: problems and plans.' *In* Connolly, K. J. (Ed.) *Mechanisms of Motor Skill Development.* London/New York: Academic Press.

—— (1973) 'Factors influencing the learning of manual skills by young children.' *In* Hinde, R. A., Stevenson-Hinde, J. (Eds.) *Constraints on Learning.* London/New York: Academic Press.

Elliott, J., Connolly, K. (1974) 'Hierarchical organisation in skill development.' *In* Connolly, K. J., Bruner, J. S. (Eds.) *The Growth of Competence.* London/New York: Academic Press.

Evarts, E. V. (1967) 'Representation of movements and muscles by pyramidal tract neurons of the precentral motor cortex.' *In* Yahr, M. D., Purpura, D. P. (Eds.) *Neurophysiological Basis of Normal and Abnormal Motor Activities.* Hewiett, N. Y.: Raven Press.

Greene, P. H. (1973) 'Problems of organisation of motor systems.' *In* Rosen, R., Snell, R. (Eds.) *Progress in Theoretical Biology,* vol. 2. New York/London: Academic Press.

Harrison, A., Connolly, K. (1971) 'The conscious control of fine levels of neuromuscular firing in spastic and normal subjects.' *Developmental Medicine and Child Neurology,* **13,** 762.

Hefferline, R. F. (1958) 'The role of proprioception in the control of behavior.' *Transactions of the New York Academy of Sciences,* **20,** 739.

Hein, A., Held, R. (1962) 'A neural model for labile sensorimotor co-ordination.' *In* Bernard, E. E., Kare, M. R. (Eds.) *Biological Prototypes and Synthetic Systems.* New York: Plenum Press.

Holst, E. von (1954) 'Relations between the central nervous system and peripheral organs.' *British Journal of Animal Behaviour,* **2,** 89.

—— Mittelstaedt, H. (1950) 'Das Reafferenzprinzip.' *Naturwissenschaften,* **37,** 464.

Meetham, A. R. (1969) *Encyclopaedia of Linguistics, Information and Control.* Oxford/New York: Pergamon Press.

Pribram, K. H. (1971) *Languages of the Brain.* New Jersey: Prentice-Hall.

—— Kruger, L., Robinson, R., Berman, A. J. (1955) 'The effects of precentral lesions on the behavior of monkeys.' *Yale Journal of Biology and Medicine,* **28,** 428.

Sperry, R. W. (1952) 'Neurology and the mind-brain problem.' *American Scientist,* **40,** 291.

CHAPTER NINE

Observing Motor Skill: A Developmental Approach

LEWIS ROSENBLOOM and MOYA E. HORTON

During their early years children exhibit a rapidly improving quality of motor performance, and one result of this is the acquisition of a certain deftness and precision in the execution of manipulative tasks. The pattern of maturation of some of the components of this skilful manipulation is described in this study.

Many factors contribute to the quality of skilled motor performance, including intellectual ability, visuomotor function, the state of neuromuscular development and the availability of learning opportunities. However, it is the end-point of all these, the actual motor functioning, which is the subject of interest in this study. This can be illustrated by considering, for example, the simple task of placing a series of rods into holes. Each rod has to be picked up singly, manoeuvred into the appropriate grasping position, transported to its hole and released into it, and the whole series then has to be repeated a number of times. It was in respect of these components that the changes in the quality of movements executed by young children of different ages were observed. Thus, for the purpose of the study, no regard was paid to other aspects of the children's activity which would be significant in any total evaluation of their abilities or disabilities.

A review of the literature reveals that little is known of the developmental changes in skilled motor performance. This was pointed out by Munn (1965) and Connolly (1970), although the latter did emphasise the great deal of descriptive work on motor development that has been published.

One component that has been studied is speed of response. Goodenough and her co-workers (Goodenough and Brian 1929, Goodenough and Tinker 1930, Goodenough 1935) measured speed of tapping on a keyboard with a stylus and showed that there was a steady improvement with age. More recent studies of speed of performance have been made by Davol using a rotary pursuit task (Davol *et al.* 1965), while Connolly compared the speed and accuracy of performance of groups aged six, eight and ten years, on a simple target task (Connolly *et al.* 1968). A significant increase of speed was found with age, but with no similar increase in accuracy. In both studies, some improvement occurred with practice.

Another aspect of skilled motor performance that has been studied is the developmental changes that are seen in associated movements. Fog and Fog (1963) observed that there was a progressive fall in associated movements with age, while Connolly and Stratton (1968) examined the responses of children from five years upwards to a series of tests of associated movements and demonstrated the changes that are seen with increasing age.

It can be seen that studies hitherto were confined to the development of speed and accuracy and to the progressive inhibition of associated movements as components of skilled manipulative performance in children of five years and older. This resulted in two obvious gaps in knowledge in this field of child development. The first is that components of motor skill other than the ones referred to above have not been recognised and studied, and motor skill has in fact been defined in somewhat narrow terms as being revealed by deftness and accuracy in limited movement (Jones and Seashore 1944). The second gap is that the age group under five years has been virtually ignored, so that a period of very rapid motor development has remained unexplored. The reasons for this include the difficulty of finding a suitable experimental method that can consistently be applied to children under five years. In this study an attempt was made to circumvent these difficulties by a fresh analysis of the components of skill and by extending this analysis to a younger age group.

Method

Attempts to select a suitable task for study, to record it unambiguously by different observers and to analyse it, all presented some difficulties. The apparatus used in previous studies of motor ability was designed primarily for quantitative observations and resulted in activities which were repetitive and fatiguing for the children and which did not hold the children's attention for very long. Another problem encountered in attempts to obtain precise measures of motor progress was that the end result of a motor performance was often recorded rather than changes in the components of that activity.

In view of these difficulties, we decided to use observational techniques, as these would provide the opportunity of recording the qualitative changes in performance. A doll's tea-set was chosen as suitable play material because it held the attention of all children in the age range to be studied (18 months to five years) and was familiar to all children from their nursery experience. The observers' interest centred around the children's handling of a tea-pot containing water.

Clearly, a pre-requisite to the acquisition of skilled motor performance is the development of those movements necessary for its execution. Once present, these movements are used with an increasing localisation so that they become economical and appropriate. At the same time, unwanted and associated movements become progressively less obvious. For this study, the three components of movement that were observed and recorded were (1) type of grasp used, (2) the degree of proximal limb movement and (3) the degree of associated movement of the opposite limb. Three-point scales were used to delineate these observations, as shown in Table I.

Further analysis of the components of motor skill was based very approximately on the work of Laban (Laban and Lawrence 1947). In his view, motor skill can be seen as the acquisition of a sense for the correct proportionality of four inter-related elements namely, exertion, space, control and speed. The exertion appropriately utilised in any motor activity may be 'light' or 'strong', the control may be 'fluent' or 'bound', the pathway that a movement takes through space can be 'flexible' or 'direct', and the time element may be 'quick' or 'sustained'. It follows that any lack of skill in a motor activity can be assessed in terms of these four components, although such analyses have not hitherto been applied to the development of manipulative skill in young children. Observations preliminary to this study, however, revealed that young children tend to make efforts which on the whole are too fluent, too light and too flexible. The method used in this study was however unsuitable for estimating the speed of motor performance, and hence evaluation of this component was omitted from detailed consideration in the subsequent observations that were made.

For the remaining three components (exertion, control and space), four-point descriptive scales were devised, based on children's lifting and pouring from a toy tea-pot. These scales are given in Table II.

Fifty-seven children (24 boys, 33 girls) took part in this study. The age range was from one year five months to four years eight months, giving a mean age of three years five months.

The children were attending either a day nursery or a nursery school. Each child was seen on one occasion, and in effect, therefore, profiles of manipulative behaviour of individual children within this age range were studied.

In the experimental situation, each child's ability in lifting and pouring from a toy tea-pot containing water, was studied. One child only was observed at any one time, although the children usually played in groups of two. Observation took place with the child sitting at a table at elbow height. There was a 'Galt' child's tea-set on the table, the tea-pot of which is approximately 15 cm high. This tea-pot was kept filled to a specific level so that its weight was, on average, about 400 gm, and could be lifted easily by the youngest and smallest child (see Fig. 1).

A nursery assistant was available to initiate or direct play as necessary, and each child was given a few minutes to become accustomed to the playthings (although all children had had much experience of this type of play in their nursery environments). After this initial period, each child was observed for ten minutes by two observers viewing through a one-way screen. At the end of this practice period, recording of the grade achieved in each of the six components of skill referred to above was made independently by each of the observers, on a prepared proforma.

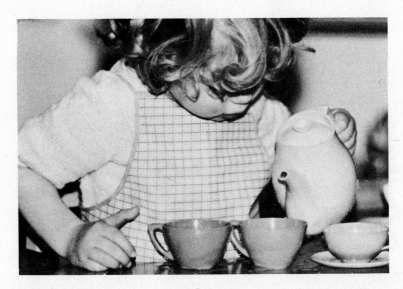

Fig. 1.

113

TABLE I

CRITERIA OF THE THREE-POINT SCALES USED IN THE OBSERVATIONS ON APPROPRIATE USE OF MOVEMENTS

Situation: Lifting toy teapot and pouring from it.

1. *Appropriateness of grasp*

   Grade 3. Teapot lifted by handle with grasping and steadying action of fingers and thumb.
   Grade 2. Teapot lifted by handle with grasping, but without steadying action.
   Grade 1. Teapot lifted by grasping body rather than handle, using one or both hands.
   Note: In grades 2 and 3, the teapot is sometimes intermittently supported by the child putting a second hand round the body of the vessel.

2. *Degree of proximal movement of limb used in pouring*

   Grade 3. Predominantly elbow/radio-ulnar movement.
   Grade 2. Predominantly shoulder movement.
   Grade 1. Presence of trunk movement.

3. *Associated movements of opposite limb to that used in lifting and pouring*

   Grade 3. No associated movement.
   Grade 2. Small associated movements.
   Grade 1. Large associated (mirror) movements.

TABLE II

CRITERIA OF THE FOUR-POINT SCALES USED IN THE OBSERVATIONS ON APPROPRIATE USE OF EFFORT

Situation: Lifting toy teapot and pouring from it.

1. *Exertion*

   Grade 4. Teapot lifted with one hand and maintained upright prior to pouring.
   Grade 3. Teapot lifted with one hand but tilted from upright prior to pouring action.
   Grade 2. Both hands used to lift teapot clear of table, or with only one hand used, teapot not lifted clear.
   Grade 1. In spite of both hands used, teapot not lifted clear of surface of table.

2. *Space i.e.* pathway that movement takes.

   Grade 4. No part of teapot ever more than just vertically clear of receiver while lifting or pouring.
   Grade 3. Lowermost part of teapot lifted higher than top of receiver during lifting but not pouring.
   Grade 2. Lowermost part of teapot lifted higher than top of receiver during both lifting and pouring.
   Grade 1. Teapot describing direct course at receiver and colliding with it.

3. *Control*

   Grade 4. Normal pouring (No "wobbling" of teapot).
   Grade 3. "Wobbling" of teapot when pouring.
   Grade 2. Spout of teapot rested on receiver during pouring.
   Grade 1. Uncontrolled swaying of teapot throughout lifting and pouring.

114

TABLE III

RESULTS: APPROPRIATE USE OF MOVEMENTS

Component	Grade	Number of children in grade	Mean age of children in grade (months)	Standard deviation (months)	Observer agreement	
					No. of observations by each person	% agreement
1. *Appropriateness of grasp*					54/57	94.7
	3	42	47.7	8.4	40/43	93.1
	2	15	28.1	8.2	14/17	82.4
	1	0	—	—	—	—
2. *Degree of proximal movement*					54/57	94.7
	3	17	49.4	8.2	16/18	88.9
	2	34	41.8	12.1	32/35	91.4
	1	6	33.3	15.2	6/7	85.7
3. *Associated movements*					56/57	98.3
	3	11	49.0	8.7	11/11	100.0
	2	34	46.5	10.7	34/35	97.1
	1	12	29.1	7.8	11/12	91.7

TABLE IV

RESULTS: APPROPRIATE USE OF EFFORT

Component	Grade	Number of children in grade	Mean age of children in grade (months)	Standard deviation (months)	Observer agreement	
					No. of observations by each person	% agreement
1. *Exertion*					53/57	92.9
	4	27	51.0	6.6	26/27	96.3
	3	24	38.6	12.1	21/25	84.0
	2	6	27.2	7.8	6/9	66.7
	1	0	—	—	—	—
2. *Space*					52/57	91.2
	4	15	50.7	7.7	15/16	93.7
	3	22	46.8	9.1	20/23	86.9
	2	16	35.6	11.8	14/18	77.8
	1	4	24.0	7.7	3/5	60.0
3. *Control*					52/57	91.2
	4	5	53.2	3.2	5/6	83.3
	3	30	48.9	9.3	28/32	87.5
	2	18	36.1	8.3	15/19	79.9
	1	4	19.0	0.5	4/5	80.0

115

If more than one grade of behaviour was seen for any one component, the best grade achieved was the one scored. So far as laterality is concerned, the dominant limb performance was the one recorded. For those children whose laterality was not established, if the quality of performance was different on the two sides, the better performance was the one recorded. The amount of observer agreement was calculated for the individual grades of each component of skill studied, for each component as a whole, and for the complete study. The calculations were based on the total number of observations agreed by both observers divided by the total number of observations made for each item.

Results

Tables III and IV show the mean ages of the children in each grade of the six components studied, together with the standard deviations. The number of children in each grade and the degree of observer agreement are also indicated.

Discussion

In arriving at a definition of skill, two groups of components—the appropriate use of movement and the appropriate use of effort—have been observed and analysed in this study. There is one additonal component that has not hitherto been considered. It is likely that manipulative skill improves by a process of trial and error, with children making continuous adjustments in their method until a consistent pattern of behaviour is achieved. The development of consistency of performance may therefore be considered as an additional component of skill, so that the latter may now be more comprehensively defined as 'the appropriate use of movement, together with appropriate use of effort, together with consistency of performance'.

Returning to a consideration of the results presented in this study, one general point may first be made. Because of the design of the study, intercomponent comparisons are possible only between the most accomplished grades of behaviour of each component. This can be done because these grades represent mature varieties of each of these types of behaviour, so that no further improvement can be expected in the context of the particular situation studied. Thus the numbers of children achieving Grade 4 in each of the three effort components can be compared directly, but the numbers of children achieving the lower grades of these components cannot be so compared, as it cannot be demonstrated that, for example, Grade 2 of the exertion component represents an equivalent degree of skill to Grade 2 of the space or control components.

Coming to a consideration of the individual components, the types of grasp used are indicated in Tables I and III. It is of interest that none of these normal children lifted the tea-pot by the body rather than by the handle, although for some of the younger ones it would have been easier for them to have done this. This would appear to represent an intellectual awareness of the function of the handle together with a lack of appreciation as yet that ignoring the handle and grasping the body might be a more appropriate action. The knowledge that these particular abilities occur in this sequence might have an application in the management of children with impaired manipulative abilities.

116

It can be seen from Table III that the degree of proximal movement involved in lifting and pouring activities is less in older children than in younger ones in the age range studied here. Nevertheless, although only a small number of younger children exhibited trunk movement in this situation, more than half the group in all, including several four-year-olds, did show some excess of proximal movement, *i.e.* predominantly shoulder movement on pouring, and less than a third of the group, with a mean age not greatly different to those in Grade 2 for this component, had no excess of proximal activity. Similarly, as can be seen from Table III, and as might be expected from the previous studies referred to earlier, associated movements are far from being completely inhibited in pouring activities, even at the upper end of the age range. Indeed, most of the children did have small associated movements of the opposite limb, although only a minority of the youngest ones exhibited large mirror movements in this situation.

The development of the three effort components of exertion, space and control, as shown in Table IV, can be considered together. As with the other components, a progressive improvement with age can be seen for all three, but it is of interest and perhaps of significance also, that children appear to acquire ability in exertion earlier than in achieving an appropriate pathway through space, and both these abilities are acquired prior to full control of movements. Certainly, this is true for the most accomplished grades of these three components, and, as has been discussed earlier, the numbers of children in these grades are directly comparable.

It may be possible to explain these kinesiological findings on a functional/anatomical basis in connection with the type of muscle work involved in their execution. Thus the pattern of muscle work involved in tasks requiring an appropriate amount of exertion is concentric activity. This is the variety of isometric muscle work in which movement in opposition to an external force is produced, with the attachments of the active muscles being drawn towards each other. It can be postulated, therefore, that it is this type of muscle activity that is the first to mature in young children.

Similarly the type of muscular work involved in stabilising such proximal structures as the shoulder joint is possibly the next to mature. This is isotonic or static muscle function and involves the muscles contracting without any alteration in their length. This type of activity is essential for the reduction of unwanted proximal movements and is also needed to stabilise the muscles of a limb which is being moved through space. This, therefore, would be the second type of muscular activity to mature.

A further correlation can be drawn between a third variety of muscle function, *i.e.* eccentric activity, and the control component of skill. Eccentric activity is that variety of isometric muscle work which occurs when resistance to movement produced by an external force is needed, the attachments of the active muscles being drawn away from each other. Such activity is seen, for example, in the fore-arm and hand musculature, when fine control of pouring without swaying or wobbling of the vessel is needed, and it would appear therefore that this matures at a later stage than the other types of muscle function.

Clearly, this progressive maturation of varieties of muscular activity—shortening,

117

then stabilising, and finally lengthening activities—refers only to the muscle groups which are the prime movers in the particular actions studied.

The application of studies of this nature must lie ultimately in the provision of help for children with developmental disorders and abnormalities. In this context and in the absence of standardised tests of motor ability for very young children, the information gained from observation of children moving, in this and other studies, is of value. Such information can be used to assess the degree of difficulty that particular children experience in learning skilled motor activities. It is also of use in helping to identify specific causes of such difficulties, and it contributes, therefore, both to making short-term predictions of children's physical capabilities, and also to providing therapists with a sound basis for planning appropriate treatment schemes. A final advantage in observing very young children, as in this study, is that, as with many developmental disorders, early identification of physical difficulties together with the provision of optimum conditions for their solution, may help to prevent further unnecessary deterioration.

Summary

An observational study of the development of a number of the components that go to make up skilled manipulative performance in a group of normal children aged 17 months to four years eight months is described. A definition of skill in functional and kinesiological terms as the appropriate use of movement, together with appropriate use of effort, together with consistency of performance is derived. It is shown that even at the upper end of the age range studied here, maturation of all the components studied is often incomplete. The type of muscle work underlying some aspects of skilled performance is described, and a hypothesis on the rate of maturation of different types of muscular activity is advanced.

REFERENCES

Connolly, K. (1970) 'Skill development. Problems and plans.' *In Mechanisms of Motor Skill Development.* London: Academic Press.
—— Brown, K., Bassett, E. (1968) 'Development changes in some components of a motor skill.' *British Journal of Psychology,* **59,** 305.
—— Stratton, P. (1968) 'Developmental changes in associated movements.' *Developmental Medicine and Child Neurology,* **10,** 49.
Davol, S. H., Hastings, M. L., Klein, D. A. (1965) 'The effect of age, sex, and speed of rotation on rotary pursuit performance by young children.' *Perceptual and Motor Skills,* **21,** 351.
Fog, E., Fog, M. (1963) 'Cerebral inhibition examined by associated movements.' *In* Bax, M., Mac Keith, R. C. (Eds.) *Minimal Cerebral Dysfunction.* Clinics in Developmental Medicine, no. 10. London: Spastics International Medical Publications with Heinemann Medical.
Goodenough, F. L. (1935) 'A further study of speed of tapping in early childhood.' *Journal of Applied Psychology,* **19,** 309.
—— Brian, C. R. (1929) 'Certain factors underlying the acquisition of motor skill by pre-school children.' *Journal of Experimental Psychology,* **12,** 27.
—— Tinker, M. A. (1930) 'A comparative study of several methods of measuring finger tapping in children and adults.' *Journal of Genetic Psychology,* **38,** 146.
Jones, H. E., Seashore, E. H. (1944) 'The development of fine motor and mechanical abilities.' 43rd Yearbook, Part I (N.S.S.E.) Chicago: Univesity of Chicago Press.
Laban, R., Lawrence, F. C. (1947) *Effort.* London: Macdonald and Evans.
Munn, N. L. (1965) *The Evolution and Growth of Human Behaviour,* 2nd ed. London: Harrap.

RECORDING CHILDREN'S MOVEMENTS

CHAPTER TEN

Recording Children's Movements: The Development of an Observational Method

H. LORNA BRAND and P. ROSENBAUM

We have been interested in the hypothesis that lack of early mobility affects development generally and in particular restricts early learning. In order to carry out studies to test this hypothesis, it is necessary to be able to measure and record movements made by the child. We failed to find any existing system which was suitable for our purpose, nor did we find any normative data on this subject. In this paper we describe our attempts to devise a suitable system.

We decided that the system we needed should have the following characteristics:
(a) be simple and brief;
(b) be applicable in a clinical setting;
(c) show whether children move, by how much and in what way;
(d) show the purpose of movement.

The last criterion proved difficult. Initially we classified the purposes of movement as physical, intellectual, and social, together with a category of inhibition of movement. We soon found, however, that allocation to one or other of these categories was based upon personal inferences rather than upon unbiased, objective observations. Furthermore, we found that we each inferred differently on an appreciable number of occasions. In view of the warning by Holt and Reynell (1970) about the dangers of inference in this type of observation, we decided to abandon this criterion, and to restrict ourselves to observing and recording whole body movements.

The methods of Hutt *et al.* (1963), designed for use with hyperactive children, were reviewed as possibly being suitable for our purposes. They standardised the room arrangement and laid numbered squares on the floor. Trained observers recorded, in a telegrammatic way, all the movements of a child as he was actually making them. They were able to determine how long a child spent on various activities, and could make diagrams to show the distances and directions of a child's movements. Using this method they compared the amounts of activity shown by children receiving various medications. They also studied children's responses to distracting and novel stimuli by introducing new objects into the 'standard' room. However, we found this highly detailed and rather elaborate technique difficult to carry out and felt we needed an easier method for our purposes. Their work did, however, lead us to standardise our own room, and to remember their use of tape recorders when we ran into our own problem of trying to record directly onto paper.

Having decided to restrict our observations to whole body movements, we classified these into two categories which we called 'static' and 'dynamic'. The 'static' category included the basic starting position and any variation of these positions on the spot. The 'dynamic' category meant whole body displacement from one space to another space as the observation was taking place. All the possible positions and movements of a young child were identified and classified (see Fig. 1). Using this grouping and method was not always easy, and much practice was required in order to obtain a 90 per cent inter-observer reliability.

Recording directly onto paper was soon found to be difficult and unreliable, and was abandoned. We used tape recorders, and then immediately following the observation period we transcribed the recordings onto score sheets using a simple coding system we devised. Finally, we decided to base our observations upon a time sampling method. Each child was observed for 10 non-consecutive minutes during which any movements made at five-second intervals were reported and recorded.

Illustrative Example

We studied movements of normal children aged from 9 to 26 months. The children, mostly with their mothers and in groups of two or three, played in a large room, well equipped with large and small toys, chairs and tables, and a climbing frame. The mothers were told that the purpose of the exercise was to watch how the children moved as they played. We both watched through a one-way screen while the children played and made a total of 120 observations over ten non-consecutive minutes in each case.

Three tape recorders were used. One was prepared with a tape on which 'gong' sounds had been recorded at five-second intervals, and also the full minute was similarly recorded distinctively. Each observer recorded his observations onto his own hand-held tape recorder. An observation was made each time the gong sound occurred, and at the end of a full minute attention was switched to another child. Immediately at the end of each session the observations were transcribed onto a prepared sheet and any observer differences were noted.

Scoring was based upon two elements of movement. Each child was given an 'over-all' score and a 'dynamic' score. The 'over-all' score was the *total* number of position changes and was a score derived by analysing consecutive pairs of observations in the 'static' category and by tallying the number of observations in the 'dynamic' category. In any situation in which consecutive observations within a particular minute were not within the same section of the 'static' category the child was given credit for a change of position. He was also given credit for each observation in the 'dynamic' category, regardless of whether consecutive observations were in the same section of that category or not. Thus the 'dynamic' score was simply extracted from the 'over-all' score.

A typical record of one minute's period of observations is shown in Fig. 1. This figure shows the observations made during the seventh minute. Each observation is numbered. There were eight dynamic movements during this period and 11 changes of position. The changes of position were calculated as follows—

$$1 - 2 - 3 - 4$$
$$|$$
$$5 - 6 - 7 - 8 - 9 - 10 - 11$$
$$|$$
$$12$$

Name . L.D. . . . .   Date of birth .2. .10. .70. . . . .   Age 26 months . . . . .

	STATIC POSTURES							DYNAMIC MOVEMENTS										
	Lying	Kneel	Sitting floor	Sitting chair	Stand	Squat	Bend	Roll	Crawl	Mobile sit	Shuffle on spot	Walk	Run	Step	Cruise	Jump	Climb	Fall
1																		
2																		
3																		
4																		
5																		
6																		
7				5	4, 11	12						1,2,6,7, 10		3,8,9,				
8																		
9																		
10																		

Fig. 1. Score sheet showing movements recorded during seventh minute.

121

Thus there were ten changes of position. There was no change from '4' to '5' or from '11' to '12' because these were changes of static posture without change of position. Of the ten changes, eight were in the 'dynamic' category and so the 'over-all/dynamic' score for this period would be 10/8.

The results on ten normal children are shown in Fig. 2. Out of a possible 120 changes of position, these children's 'over-all' scores ranged from 21 to 78 and their 'dynamic' scores ranged from eight to 48. Whether a child moved a lot or very little, there appeared to be a ratio of approximately two to one between the number of changes of position and the number of times the child was observed to be moving.

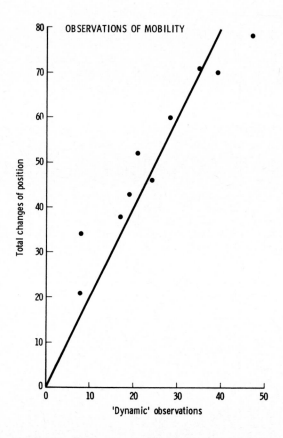

Fig. 2. Observation of movements of ten normal children.

These preliminary observations are presented to show that the method is easy to use, inexpensive to set up and has a number of potential applications. It will be very interesting to apply this technique to children with impaired mobility, and it could be used to measure changes of mobility level after a period of therapy. This method

122

could certainly be used clinically to assess the effect of various therapy regimes on the behaviour of hyperkinetic children.

REFERENCES

Holt, K. S., Reynell, J. K. (1970) *Observation of Children*. London: National Association for Mental Health.
Hutt, C., Hutt, S. J., Ounsted, C. (1963) 'A method for the study of children's behaviour.' *Developmental Medicine and Child Neurology*, **5**, 233.

CHAPTER ELEVEN

Movement Notations and the Recording of Normal and Abnormal Movements

M. HORTON and J. MCGUINNESS

When the Russians recently staged a production of Fokine's sixty-year-old ballet *Petrushka* in Moscow, they found that although most of the ballet could be reconstructed, no-one could remember Petrushka's cell dance. The Russians appealed to London for help, and a score of the Fokine choreography in Benesh movement notation was sent to a correspondence student in Moscow, who then read it to the ballet-master of the Bolshoi Ballet Company. The story is a good illustration of the remarkable fact that only in comparatively recent times has the world of ballet emerged from its oral tradition.

It seemed obvious that a movement notation would ultimately develop in a subject such as ballet, where there is a great need for accurate recording and communication.

In Britain, the use of notation systems for studying movement disorders is still largely in its infancy; the various methods of physical treatment are almost entirely dependent on oral communication.

The Requirements of Movement Notations

The central problem of any notation system is that of representing on two-dimensional paper the position in three-dimensional space of each part of the body (Causely 1966). In addition to the three dimensions of space, the fourth dimension of time also has to be recorded. Ideally, one would like to produce on paper a precise record of each movement of each part of the body and the moment when it occurs.

The notation system must have a logical structure and must be composed of mutually consistent elements, so that signs and symbols can be kept to a minimum and there can be a logical development of grammatical rules. At the same time, the system must be fairly simple, so that it remains easily legible even when recording complex material. It must also be capable of being read at sight and needs to be visualised easily and readily.

The system should have sufficient scope to be capable of recording two essential facets of movement:
(1) It must be capable of modification in order to be able to cover the various forms, styles and techniques of moving (Curl 1966).
(2) It must record fine detail of position and movement in every part of the body.

In order to fulfil these conditions, the notation needs to be sufficiently detailed to avoid ambiguity, yet not so complicated as to be unduly cumbersome.

Two systems which have gained wide acceptance are the Laban notation (which Laban called *Kinetography*) and the Benesh movement notation.

The Laban Notation

In the 1930s Rudolph Laban propounded a system of recording movement by written symbols. During the succeeding 40 years, this system has been subject to considerable modification and development. One of the new methods of using kinetographic symbols is called *Motif writing* (Preston-Dunlop 1970). The Motif system gives the outline of movement only and is proving to be a useful vehicle for describing movement in which the creative invention of the mover is of prime importance.

The Benesh Notation

Joan and Rudolf Benesh, working in London, developed a movement notation which fulfilled all the requirements described above. There now exists an Institute of Choreology and a college, to teach, provide examinations and define standards. Movement notators (choreologists) now work in the fields of ballet, physical education, work study assessment and, most recently, medicine. The Benesh notation is the one now being used clinically, and as one of us (Julia McGuinness) has considerable experience of its clinical application, this method will be described in greater detail.

The Benesh notation is based on the science of linear perspective, *i.e.* the manner in which the eye and brain see and translate three dimensions into two on the retina and back again. The notation is written on a five-line stave and reads from left to right. The human figure is imposed on this stave in an upright position, viewed from the back (see Fig. 1). The notator is trained to read from top to bottom of the stave at any given moment in time (shown along the stave) and is therefore able to incorporate all the information of that moment at a glance.

Three signs are used to denote the placing of the extremities in space. The language of the notation defines the extremity as the extreme point of the limb—either the arm or the leg. These three signs are:

      — in space, level with the body
      | in space, in front of the body
      • in space, behind the body

By manipulating these signs to form crosses, three further signs are developed to indicate the positions of the joints:

      ⊹ in space, level with the body
      ┼ in space, in front of the body
      ✕ in space, behind the body

Figures 2 and 3 show the use of these basic signs in the stave.

Limb movement is shown by *movement lines*. These trace the path of the moving limb from one salient point to another; they are written in or under the stave and pass through time as they are read from left to right (see Fig. 4).

The information bracketed under *a* shows a static position with the hands on the hips, hips internally rotated, knees flexed and in contact, and a wide base with the centre of gravity evenly distributed. The line at *b* indicates that a jump is taking place off both feet, while the right foot is in the air in front of the body, with full knee extension. Notation at *c* shows the landing position on left leg, with external rotation and flexion of left hip and the right leg remaining in the same position as in the jump. The position at *d* shows the legs returning to the static position.

Figure 5 shows the gait pattern of a hemiplegic patient. The information bracketed under *a* shows the static posture prior to ambulation, i.e. side flexion of head to compensate for side flexion of upper torso; displacement of shoulder girdle; spinal flexion, adduction and internal hip rotation; ankle displacement in plantar flexion; width of base; hand postures; elbow flexion and shoulder abduction. The parallel lines above *b* show the path of the left foot through the swing phase; abnormal knee contact is shown at *c*, and *d* shows the final part of swing phase and double support phase, including depth of gait and abnormal flexion of right foot.

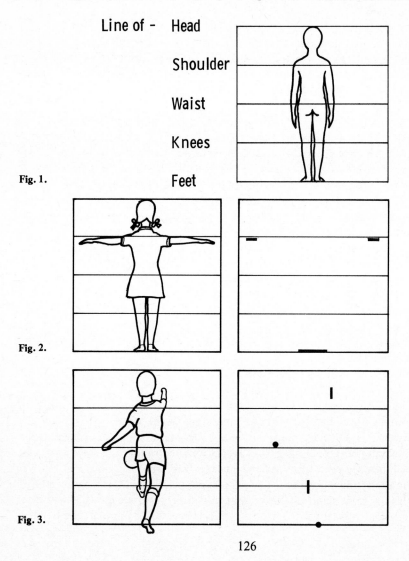

Line of - Head

Shoulder

Waist

Knees

Fig. 1.   Feet

Fig. 2.

Fig. 3.

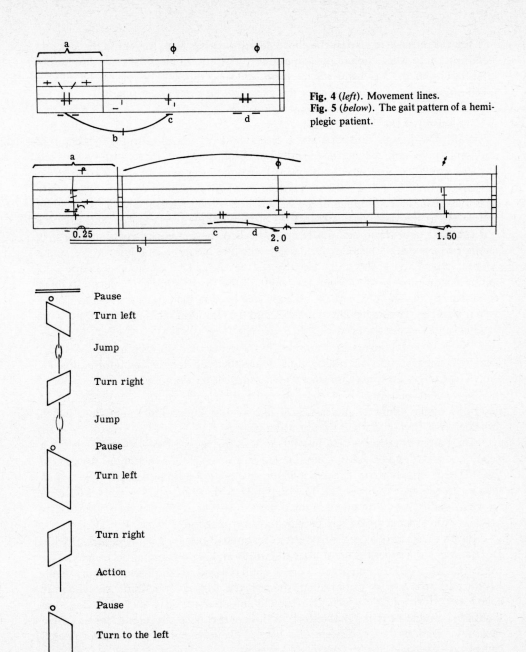

Fig. 4 (*left*). Movement lines.
Fig. 5 (*below*). The gait pattern of a hemi-plegic patient.

Pause
Turn left

Jump

Turn right

Jump

Pause

Turn left

Turn right

Action

Pause

Turn to the left

Pause

Turn to the right

Fig. 6. A staff of Laban notation read from below upwards (from Preston-Dunlop 1970).

127

For the purpose of clarity, the above description has been limited to the legs and feet during only one section of the gait pattern, whereas, in fact, the stave also carries information on the following: torso; head and arm movements; centre of gravity; speed of gait; and the remainder of the gait through right swing phase.

A Comparison of the Two Systems

Both the Laban and Benesh notation systems cope with the problem of developing a two-dimensional shape into a three-dimensional space. Both systems use a stave similar to that used in music notation, although Benesh is simpler to understand than Laban. The Benesh system uses a five-line stave which is divided into bars to indicate time. The lines of the stave intersect the body (see Fig. 1). The Laban system places the stave vertically instead of horizontally (see Fig. 6). This use of a vertical stave appears to be an attempt to record the movements of the body in a manner which readily helps us to identify with the mover in our mind's eye. Some writers have termed this our 'kinaesthetic image'. The continuous centre line represents the passage of time and the length of the symbols indicates the duration of an action. By placing the parts of the body side by side, simultaneous actions can be seen to occur at the same moment in time, and the temporal relationships between the actions can be easily deduced.

While Benesh conveys information by the particular positioning of the signs, Laban, in contrast, uses definite symbols which themselves carry the information. (It is also true to say that *some* information is gained from the position of the symbol.)

Movement pathways are recorded quite differently in the two systems. As described earlier, Benesh makes skilful use of a series of movement lines which indicate a position only when that position changes.

The Laban notation system has no symbols for the positions of the body, as a position is regarded as a movement that has come to rest and is thought of in terms of the different directions in space which the parts of the body occupy. The Laban system, therefore, emphasises action, and this is done by placing strokes—action strokes—in the stave. Movement in the three dimensions of space is then indicated by an elaboration of the action stroke which gives it a shape.

Both systems have a good descriptive vocabulary for recording dynamics, rhythm and quality of movement. Benesh uses the words and expression marks of music, for example, 'lento' (slow) 'moderato' (at a moderate pace) and 'presto' (very fast). Laban indicates quality of movement by using a simple three-dimensional figure called an 'effort graph', which gives over a hundred variants and rhythmic combinations. It must be noted that 'effort' in this context does not refer to force. Laban saw motor skill as the acquisition of a correct proportionality of four inter-related categories—exertion, space, control and speed.

Clinical Applications of the Benesh Notation System

In the 1960s Professor Milani Comparetti and Dr. E. Gidoni (1968) developed a method of assessing the movement patterns of cerebral palsied patients. The method was called 'motorscopic' examination and consisted of the following observations. (1) Spontaneous postures and motor behaviour observed systematically.

128

(2) Movements performed following instructions from the examiner.

(3) Movement patterns under certain stimulus situations.

To record these motorscopic patterns, a suitable recording method was needed which would enable the information to be processed, measured and analysed for clinical and research purposes.

A grant from the United Cerebral Palsy Research and Educational Foundation enabled a choreologist to work at Professor Milani's clinic for one year. During the year, notation records were made of 100 normal babies, 17 normal adults and 93 cerebral palsied children, aged from 9 months to 15 years. About 5000 patterns of posture and movement were notated, using the following situations:

(a) routine developmental testing of babies;

(b) training classes for physiotherapy students;

(c) cerebral palsied children in daily-life activities and during assessment sessions with a physiotherapist;

(d) movements of patients and therapists during Temple-Fay, Bobath and proprio-ceptive neuro-muscular facilitation methods.

The results of the study showed that the Benesh system was an effective tool for recording both normal and abnormal movement patterns. Also, it was shown that complex data could be incorporated on a single page of clinical records and in this way could be used for future reference. Previously, one had to rely on inadequate verbal description, two-dimensional photographs, or memory.

No matter what form of pathological movement is being recorded, the notation remains wholly objective. Its comprehensive vocabulary covers all postures (prone, supine, side-lying, sitting), forms of mobility and all dynamics, rhythms and qualities of movement.

It is worth pointing out that although the movement patterns of a muscular dystrophy patient might well have the same notation in the stave as that of a spastic cerebral palsied patient, the use of dynamic, rhythmic and timing signs written above the stave will indicate the fact that the movements are in fact the antithesis of each other.

One of the many advantages of using notation systems is that the notator (choreologist) can remain quite apart from the subject without interfering in any way or having any effect on results. One example which illustrates this point is found in the field of ergonomics. Information as to how people sat in various types of arm-chairs was collected by placing the chairs in a hotel lobby, where the choreologist sat in a suitable viewing position and worked unnoticed (Kember et al. 1972).

In contrast, the use of film and video techniques usually involves interference with the physician/patient relationship, and the moving around of electrical equipment thus creates a somewhat artificial atmosphere. The two-dimensional information must further be transposed into some form of notation (written notes, graphs etc. . .) to be of any value.

In addition to enabling one to see retrospective information at a glance, the Benesh system also provides a method of quick comparative analysis. This method— called the 'transparency technique'—is in fact very simple.

For example, Fig. 7 shows a child attempting to walk with calipers and crutches; Fig. 8 shows the same child's attempts three months later. If Fig. 7 is written in red ink and Fig. 8 written in black ink on a transparent sheet, then by laying one on top of the other, information regarding the differences between the two recordings is immediately available.

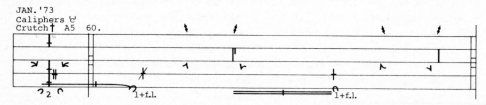

Fig. 7

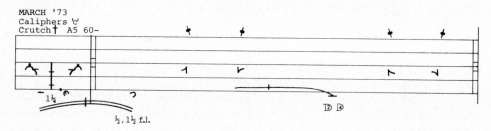

Fig. 8

Conclusions

The suitability of notation systems for recording movement depends precisely on what one wishes to observe. The spatio-temporal aspects of movement present no recording difficulties, but the subtleties of the more complex aspects of human movement are not always assessed. Just as language does not record accent and intonation, so it is with notation, and yet it is these aspects which concern us most when recording the problems of a child with physical difficulties. In the clinical world, observation is carried out with treatment in mind and is directed to what is causing or producing a movement. The clinician will want to discover, for example, how a child with involuntary movements copes with them, or whether an abnormal gait is caused by musculo-skeletal difficulties. More experience of notation systems is required in order to discover fully their potential for detailed assessment and analysis.

Claims are made that notation is a tool for analysis. This is certainly so, in the sense that anything which forces one to think systematically about a subject can be described as such.

The notation systems are capable of modification to meet the requirements of different disciplines. In a sense, the more disciplines which adopt them, the richer they become. Specialists in one area make greater use of certain aspects, but the basic notation of one system can be used by many disciplines. In notating hand function, for example, the whole of the Benesh stave can be re-labelled a hand stave, with each line representing one finger. However, just as with a map, if one wants greater details of one area, one must sacrifice the map as a whole, so with some adaptation of the notation, one would need to sacrifice certain information.

While it is true that annotation of movement is open to similar objections as other observation techniques, there is certainly a gain in objectivity. Ambiguities of recording are generally absent, although the extent to which this is achieved depends on the skill of the observer. Just as in listening to music some can appreciate only intervals of semitones and others can appreciate ranges in between, so the same differences in appreciation can exist in movement notation.

Concluding Remarks

In the field of child development, notation systems could be used with advantage to enrich and discipline observation methods, to provide reliable material on which to base re-education programmes, and to provide a more detailed picture of the way developing children use movement. This, one hopes, would lead to a greater understanding of the needs of the handicapped.

Summary

Movement notation is an objective recording tool. Experiences with the Benesh system show that movement notation has many uses in the medical field, where clear, accurate and detailed records of motor skills are required, and where a vast amount of information is needed for comparative analysis. Experience of notation can enrich and discipline observation methods.

Acknowledgements

Fig. 6 was taken from *Readers in Kinetography, Laban Series B, Book I,* by P. Preston-Dunlop, and was reproduced by kind permission of Macdonald and Evans Ltd.

REFERENCES

Causley, M. (1966) *An Introduction to Benesh Movement Notation. Its General Principles and its Use in Physical Education.* London: Parrish.

Curl, G. F. (1966) *An Enquiry into Movement Notation,* Part I. London: Chelsea College of Education.

Milani Comparetti, A., Gidoni, E. A. (1968) 'A graphic method of recording normal and abnormal movement patterns.' *Developmental Medicine and Child Neurology,* **10,** 633.

Kember, P. A., Shackel, B., Branton, P. (1972) *A Preliminary Field Study of Sitting, Comfort and Easy Chairs with a New Observation Method.* MSc Thesis. Loughborough University of Technology.

Preston-Dunlop, V. (1970) *Readers in Kinetography—Laban.* 2nd ed. *Series B.* London: Macdonald and Evans.

CHAPTER TWELVE

Objective Methods and Implications of Recording Children's Behaviour

M. J. MACCULLOCH

Child psychiatry is probably the least structured of the medical arts. There are two reasons for this: first, because of its traditions, which perhaps rest too firmly on psychoanalytic interests and dogma; and second, because of its inherent difficulties, which stem from the multiplicity of causes of disordered behaviour in the child.

In order to arrive at a diagnostic formulation in the case of a psychiatrically disturbed child it is necessary to consider the following factors:
(1) the physiological development status of the child;
(2) the child's personality;
(3) the child's learning history;
(4) the parents' personalities;
(5) the interaction of the child's personality with the parents' personalities;
(6) the interactions of the child with his peers and teachers;
(7) any specific relevant stress demands on the child;
(8) any current acute or chronic medical condition of the CNS (or other systems).

Such a diagnostic formulation (the logical prerequisite to treatment) is assisted by a developmental history taken from the child's mother, together with details of the child's current behaviour. The child's behaviour is then observed on several occasions and his performance on psychometric tests is assessed. That there exists genuine difficulty in assessing and diagnosing behavioural/psychological disorders can be illustrated by reference to studies on the incidence of behavioural disorders. For instance, the Underwood Committee (1955) suggested that between 5.4 and 9.7 per cent of the population showed behavioural disturbances, while Ullman (1952) found an incidence rate of eight per cent.

Mitchell and Shepherd (1966) studied a random sample of one in ten children aged between five and 15 years, using ratings made by both parents and teachers. They found that of the 6077 children studied, ten per cent were rated by parents or teachers as having three or more marked behavioural problems, but only one in five of this sample was picked out on both questionnaires as falling in the worst ten per cent of the total number of children studied. This discrepancy clearly highlights the difficulty that besets child psychiatric diagnosis.

Similarly, Rutter and Graham (1966) studied 2193 children who were born on the Isle of Wight between 1 September 1953 and 31 August 1955. They found there was a minimum prevalence rate of 6.3 per cent for children with behavioural disorders (excluding those suffering from mental subnormality), 2.2 per cent of the children being classed as having severe behavioural disorders. Of this 6.3 per cent, 36

132

per cent showed neurotic behaviour, 32 per cent antisocial disorders, 22 per cent mixed disorders, 5 per cent developmental habit disorders, 1.5 per cent childhood psychoses, 1.5 per cent hyperkinetic syndrome, and 2 per cent personality deviations. In addition, 2.6 per cent (57) of the population of 2193 were identified as being intellectually retarded and 85 showed a 28-month retardation in reading, using a multiple regression approach to take into account intellectual level and chronological age (Rutter *et al.* 1972).

The difficulties of classification may be further illustrated by reference to the example of hyperkinesis.

Hyperactivity has been defined by Werry *et al.* (1968) as a *chronic, sustained, excessive level of motor activity which is the cause of significant complaint both at home and at school.* Chess (1960) has pointed out that hyperkinesis is *one of the most common manifestations of disturbed childhood behaviour.* She found that ten per cent of the children seen in her private practice were referred directly for hyperactivity, and Patterson *et al.* (1971) found this to be the commonest referral symptom in four child guidance clinics. Similarly, Stewart *et al.* (1966) give an estimated incidence rate of hyperkinesis of four per cent of all school-age children, and Ounsted (1955) found that of a group of 830 epileptic children, eight per cent were hyperactive. Using an interdisciplinary approach, Kenny *et al.* (1971) reported on the examination of 100 children referred on account of hyperactivity, with three examiners taking part in each case. In 299 separate clinical examinations of these children, hyperactivity was judged to be present in only 75. More than half of the children were not considered to be hyperactive by any of the examiners, and one third were judged to be hyperactive by the majority. There was no close agreement among the examiners on whether hyperactivity was or was not present.

A leader in the *British Medical Journal* eloquently amplified the problem (1973, *Vol.* I, p. 305):

'The specific learning difficulties which these children with minimal cerebral dysfunction encounter put them under increased stress at school, and in consequence they are likely to suffer from secondary emotional disturbance, which aggravates their hyperactivity. Apart from this, emotional disturbance as such in children can arise from a wide range of other causes in the school and in the home and express itself as hyperactivity. Having only one parent in the family, parental alcoholism, drug addiction, parental criminality, parent-child conflicts, sibling rivalry, abnormal fears, anti-social tendencies, repression at school, inadequate school performance, disturbance occasioned by an inappropriate education milieu, and cultural inadequacy can all contribute to emotional disturbance in children. Lastly, the child with mental defect and a limited ability to understand, to concentrate, and to occupy his mind may pass much of his time in aimless hyperactivity. Drugs...may result in striking improvement, though their effect on the individual child is difficult to predict.'

However, although there is a general agreement as to the existence of the hyperactive syndrome as a major childhood disorder, there has been little work on the reliable measurement of the dependent variables (*e.g.* activity level, attention span, visuo-motor deficit *etc.*) and it should be noted that early diagnosis may lead to a better prognosis for such children (Stewart *et al.* 1966). In the case of activity level in particular, subjective ratings are still the usual mode of assessment and it is worth quoting Werry *et al.* (1968) at length:

'However . . . . . . the methodology of most studies leaves much to be desired, particularly in the absence of a control group, statistical analysis of data, and precise and reliable measures. Since the time of Grant's review (1962) the use of a placebo group is certainly more common, but the techniques of measurement of the dependent variables, such as activity level and aggressiveness, have shown little, if any substantial improvement, particularly in the use of direct rather than differential, and atomistic rather than global, techniques.'

It will be seen from this brief review that there is genuine difficulty in measuring hyperkinetic behaviour. It logically follows that any system which can contribute to any part of this chain of diagnostic events and which increases the reliability of our observations will increase therapeutic efficiency. The first part of our solution to this problem—that of objective measures of childhood behaviour—is now described. A highly promising apparatus, known as a Human Automated Two Subject Open Field (HATSOF), for measuring total body movement over a room area has been described by MacCulloch *et al.* (1969). This is a novel and sophisticated electro-mechanical device which provides data in the form of an eight-channel punch-paper tape.

In Birmingham we sought to create an environment which would reliably measure behaviour and permit experimentation on behaviour change. It seemed most feasible to measure spatial position in a room, for such a system would permit experimentation (*e.g.* by changing the objects in the room) and the subject might be capable of recording his own spatial position by his physical presence. A measuring system was required which would fulfil two major criteria: first, and most important, the data generated should be 'hard' *i.e.* irrefutable; and second, the primary observation technique should require minimal manipulation of the subjects. A third, but scarcely less important consideration, was system capacity. It was felt that measurements such as the distance covered by the child and details of track could be massively tedious and therefore automated data acquisition was thought to be mandatory.

Such specifications ruled out paper-and-pencil techniques, filming, video-tape techniques, and subject-attached devices such as telemeters, pedometers and the like. Two approaches for recording a free subject in two planes suggested themselves: first, to render the above floor space sensitive by using pairs of light sources and photo cells; and second, to render the floor itself subject-sensitive. It was suggested by Grant (1968) that the simultaneous recording of two subjects (rather than one) would be immensely rewarding in terms of data and its possible interpretation. Accordingly, we chose to render the floor sensitive in such a way as to enable the data recorder to differentiate two tracks, and so that the following combinations of experimental observations could be made: infant/infant; infant/child; infant/adult; child/child; child/adult; adult/adult.

Several methods of subject differentiation were considered and all involved the nature of the shoes worn by the subject: one constant parameter was obviously weight, which could be used in all cases except for very light infants. Therefore a weight-sensitive system was a mandatory choice, and the floor was also required to consist of appropriately small discrete areas. Sequential triggering of these areas (or tiles) formed the basis for logging movement in terms of distance, speed, and actual spatial track. The identification of the second subject by use of conducting shoe soles (to short and exposed twin metal coil on the tile surface, or to de-tune sub-tile circuits) was abandoned, and instead, each tile was fitted with reed switches which were activated by strong magnets fitted in the heels of special plastic 'playroom' shoes. Thus the system *in toto* will be seen to consist of three components:

(1) the peripheral subject-sensitive tiles;
(2) a space and time encoder;
(3) a decoder and calculator (in this case a KDF.9 computer).

The first two component parts will now be specified in brief.

(1) The Two-Subject-Sensitive Floor

A room 17 feet by 11 feet (5.18m by 3.3m) was used as the experimental space. This was overlooked, via a one-way screen, from an adjoining room suitable for the installation of the necessary electronic and electro-mechanical equipment.

The experimental room was fitted with a sub-floor one inch (2.54cm) thick and this was then used to suspend 156 wooden tiles 12 inches (30.48cm) square by 0.5 inches (1.27cm) thick. The suspension was tripartite, and consisted of: (a) four foam-rubber discs, one inch (2.54cm) in diameter which absorbed a light impact of about 20lb (9kg), (b) firm, but slightly compressible rubber cylinders which took a load of up to 60lb (27.18kg), and (c) heavy hard-rubber cylinders, diameter one inch (2.54cm) which could take a load up to 80lb (36.24kg). The suspension was arranged as in Fig. 1.

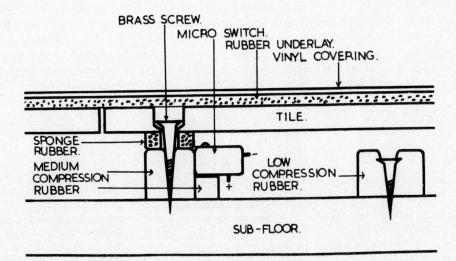

Fig. 1. Elevation view of a tile showing suspension and pressure microswitch.

135

The Switches

Four micro-switches were mounted on 0.5in (1.27cm) high, medium compression rubber cylinders using rubber cement. The suspension was so arranged that the tile deflection required to close a switch was 1/16in; the soft rubber mountings under the switches ensured that the micro-switch bodies remained undamaged under very high loads.

Sixteen reed switches were cemented to the underside of each tile: their spatial arrangement and that of the microswitch and rubber mountings are shown in Fig. 2.

Electrical Connections to the Floor

The two types of switch attached to each tile were connected in parallel sets so that each tile was served by one set of four micro-switches in parallel and one set of sixteen reed switches in parallel. Each set of switches then formed one composite switch monitoring the whole tile. The data encoder (see next section) was designed to scan the state of the tile switches every 0.2 sec and punch that information on to an eight-hole paper tape. This operation required that the floor data be reduced to its minimal form and this process was achieved by arranging the tile outputs so that, on activation of a tile, a current flowed in lines representing the row and the column appropriate to the position of the tile on the floor. This arrangement allowed specific information about the state of a tile switch to be inferred from data on the current flowing in the row and column lines (Fig. 3).

(2) The Data Encoder (Fig. 4)

The purpose of the data encoder was to put the information gained from the floor area into a form suitable for storage (on paper tape) so that it could be processed later by a digital computer. The incoming information consisted of pulses distributed in both time and space, and in order to describe the original system in full (subject space-time interrelations) it was necessary to record both these parameters. The most economical method of recording this type of information is to sample each of the lines in a predetermined sequence. The temporal information is stored by sampling at a fixed rate, enabling the time of occurrence of an event to be determined by 'counting' the number of samples taken before that event. The details of the type of event which occur are contained in the code combination punched on to the paper tape.

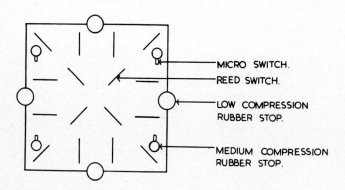

MICRO SWITCH.

REED SWITCH.

LOW COMPRESSION RUBBER STOP.

MEDIUM COMPRESSION RUBBER STOP.

Fig. 2. Plan view of single tile showing spatial arrangement of suspension, pression-sensitive micro-switches and magnet-sensitive reed switches.

136

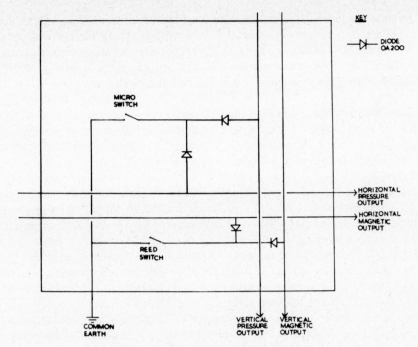

Fig. 3. Wiring and output from a single tile.

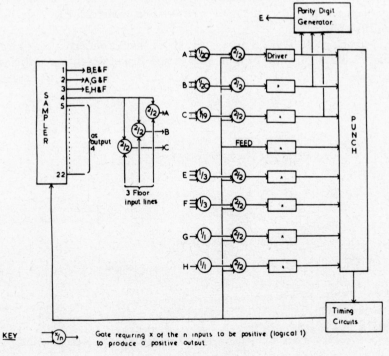

Fig. 4. The data encoder.

137

The code employed is the standard Friden Flexowriter Code. The information is stored as a series of binary-coded octal numbers by grouping the row and column outputs from the floor in threes, thus providing eight possible combinations. Each set of three floor-output lines are sampled in turn, one complete sample of the floor requiring 0.2 sec. determined by the maximum punch operating speed (110 characters/second).

The data encoder shown in Fig. 4 consists of a sampling circuit which generates a sequence of pulses used to interrogate the floor area. A train of timing pulses generated by the punch forms the input to a five-bit ripple counter, the outputs of which are decoded by means of a diode matrix providing 22 sequential outputs. Each output is positive (logical 1) for 9.1msec of the 200msec floor-sample period and no two are positive at the same time. The first three in each period drive the punch channels appropriate to the three editing characters, the driving pulses being timed to the punch operating cycle by 4.5msec timing pulses. The remaining 19 outputs each sample three floor lines in turn (28 pressure lines and 28 magnetic lines) and the states of the tile switches at the sampling instant are transferred to the punch-paper tape. The parity digit is calculated from the first three punch channels (*i.e.* those containing the floor information) which enables data errors to be detected directly, without reference to the additional channels.

The order in which the floor lines are sampled is unimportant, but by a suitable choice some degree of optimization of the following parameters may be obtained: computer programme simplicity; readability of the paper tape; and instantaneous peak power drawn from the power supply. The first and third factors are important to the design engineer and the second to the operator or psychiatrist. Fig. 5 shows a flow diagram of the floor.

Challacombe *et al.* (1972), using this device, have conducted an observation experiment on dissimilar twins of 14 months of age, one of whom was suffering from coeliac disease.

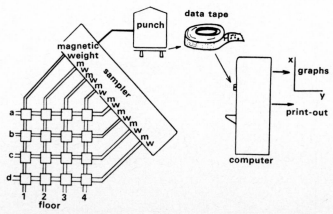

Fig. 5. Flow diagram of the floor showing the matrixed connection of the tiles (to register weight and magnetic field), the line sampler, and eight-channel data punch. The data tapes are processed off-line.

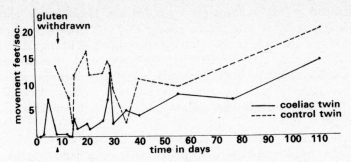

Fig. 6. A graph derived from a floor print-out showing the change-over time of exploratory behaviour in a dizygotic twin pair, one of whom is recovering from coeliac disease.

Fig. 6 demonstrates that the coeliac child was initially engaged in less exploratory movement than the twin, and that six days after gluten withdrawal the exploratory rate began to increase. Thereafter, exploration increased over the following 100 days and these trends were statistically significant. Although this study is a simple one it is an important precursor to studies that will quantify exploratory movement under differing conditions and across dissimilar groups of subjects. The way is now open, therefore, to reliably assess the effects of various drugs and other forms of treatment on children suffering from a whole range of disorders which will obviously include hyperkinesis and infantile autism. The possibility of measuring the movement of a second subject clearly suggests parent/child interaction studies and more accurate approach-avoidance work of the type reported by Currie and Brannigan (1968).

This system (HATSOF) has now been developed in a portable version of 300 ft² (91.44m²) so that it may be used at various locations such as classrooms, training centres, autistic units, and in ward areas (Birtles 1972*a*). In addition, it has had three facilities added to it, the first being hand-operated recording buttons for behavioural observations by up to ten observers working simultaneously. The second and third facilities are more significant and are therefore described in some detail.

Recording of Physiological Correlates of Exploratory Behaviour: an Automated Heart-Rate Telemeter

Telemetric methods of measurement have the advantage that the subject is fairly free to move and, more especially, parameters can be recorded in relation to time. Telemeters consist of a receiver placed in the subject's proximity and a transmitter attached to the subject—there are no direct connections between the subject and the recorder. Many uses have been made of the telemeter for monitoring biopotentials, for example, cardiac function (Longo and Pellegrino 1967), respiration (Stattleman and Cook 1966), movement of a body part (Brown and Whitman 1963), and heart and muscle output (Ko and Neuman 1967).

Birtles and Dixon (1972) have designed and built an automated heart-rate telemeter as part of our over-all behaviour logging system. Briefly, it consists of a Parks Laboratories telemeter transmitter and receiver. The ECG signal is appropriately amplified to drive a linear pen in a Bell and Howell ultraviolet recorder. Simultaneously, the signal is further processed to give a beat by beat print-out of heart rate, which is displayed on the ultraviolet polygraph. The original ECG signal is also used to drive a spare data channel on the floor data punch. The QRS-ECG signal complex is amplified and also used to drive one punch pin synchronously (to 1/110th of a second) so that the heart-rate data are encoded in analogue form on the same tape as the floor data and the observational data. The heart-rate telemeter system is shown in Fig. 7.

MacCulloch and Williams (1971) have recorded heart rates in 19 autistic and nine subnormal children and ten normal controls, using a heart-rate telemeter with cardiotachograph write-out facility. They found that heart rate was under-controlled in autistic children, in other words acceleration and deceleration were under-damped, and this finding led them to hypothesize that posterior mid-brain damage is responsible for some of the behaviour changes seen in autistic children. MacCulloch *et al.* (1971) have used the same technique and methods of analysis to measure the heart rate variance in a group of cerebral palsied children, ten of whom showed athetoid/dystonic disorder and 20 spastic cerebral disorder. The heart-rate variability expressed in standard deviation units correctly categorized seven out of the ten athetoid children and 19 of the 20 spastic children, the athetoid children having a standard deviation of heart rate above 12.00 and the spastic group having a standard

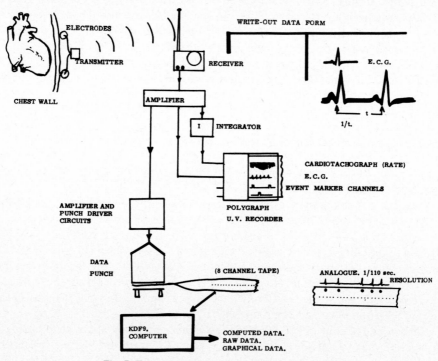

Fig. 7. Telemetered heart rate data handling system.

140

deviation of heart rate below 12.00. This second finding may have diagnostic implications for cerebral palsy and, as the authors suggest, it may also indicate at least part of the site of the damage in cerebral palsy.

A Technique for Automatically Testing Visuo-motor Performance Behaviour

Birtles *et al.* (1971) have described an off-line automated subject/machine interface which presents visuo-motor tasks to subjects and logs the results on an off-line data encoder of a type similar to that described in relation to the human open field (floor). The device, a computer-assisted psychometric system (CAPS), is shown in Fig. 8 and has been used on a group of 70 adolescent girls to assess the effect of benzodiazepine drugs on a matching-to-sample visuo-motor performance task (Sambrooks *et al.* 1972). An earlier version of the machine was used to assess visuo-motor performance deficit in child-rearing retardates (Butterworth 1970, personal communication). The CAPS is a versatile logging system which can be used to rate symptoms both in children and in adults; children's symptoms may be rated for severity by their parents.

Towards a Behavioural Data Logging System

The system now in existence consists of four components all based on computer analysis (Fig. 9).

(1) The flexowriter encodes general descriptive clinical details, including clinical opinions and diagnoses. In addition, this instrument is used to identify experimental runs on the telemeter, floor, and CAPS.

(2) The HATSOF can be used for the quantification and experimentation on many aspects of children's behaviour.

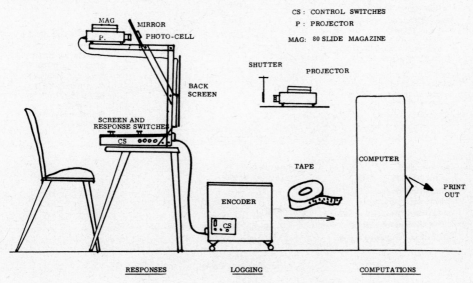

Fig. 8. Computer-assisted psychometric system.

141

(3) The HATSOF system may also be run in conjunction with the heart rate telemeter; however, the telemeter can also be used alone to record heart rate changes under various other stimulus response conditions, for example, during tasks on the CAPS.

(4) The CAPS is used in two ways: first, to take clinical behavioural histories relating to children from *both* of their parents; second, to test children's visuo-motor performance. It has a subsidiary therapeutic rôle, that of teaching matching-to-sample skills, as a precursor to reading programmes using a 'non-error' technique (Moore and Goldiamond 1964).

Data Analysis and Computation

All data tapes are given an accession number and have a tape header supplied which describes their content and indicates the programme routine to be used for their analysis. A family of data-analysing programmes is being compiled (Birtles 1972b) whereby each test or type of observation can be analysed alone. Further programmes are being written that will allow intercorrelation of various classes of data, for example to analyse the change in heart rate in relation to movement across the floor, or changes in heart rate in relation to various tasks administered by the CAPS.

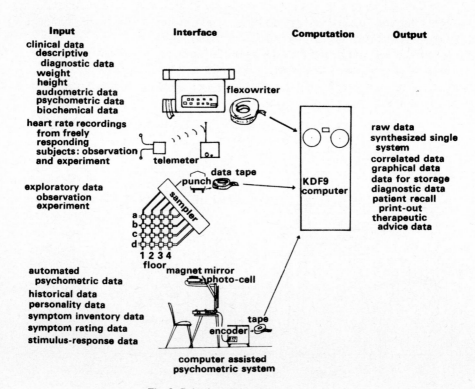

Fig. 9. Behavioural data logging system.

142

This paper describes three systems for objective measurement of aspects of behaviour in children, and the significance of measuring instruments and tools is repeatedly stressed. These tools and equipment are not ends in themselves, but follow in the long tradition of physical medicine and physiology which has made its most significant advances when new techniques and technology have been made available through the stimulus of initial observations of clinical phenomena. It is predicted that measurement of human behaviour will rapidly expand to become a sophisticated technology in the behavioural sciences and in medicine.

'I am convinced that, in experimental sciences that are evolving, and especially in those as complex as biology, discovery of a new tool for observation or experiment is much more useful than any number of systematic philosophic dissertations. Indeed, a new method or new means of investigation increases our power and makes discoveries and researches possible which would not have been possible without its help.'

Claud Bernard, 1865.

Acknowledgements

We are grateful to Ciba-Geigy for the generous provision of a Flexowriter.
It is a pleasure to acknowledge the generous support and advice given to these projects by Dr. J. Alty, K. Sharman and G. Young at the Computer Centre, Liverpool University.

REFERENCES

Birtles, C. J. (1972*a*) 'An inexpensive computer assisted psychometric system—II. The computer programs.' *International Journal of Bio-medical Computing,* 3, 223.
—— (1972*b*) Personal communication.
—— Dixon, K. (1972) Personal communication.
—— Sambrooks, J. E., MacCulloch, M. J., Holland, P. (1971) 'An inexpensive computer assisted psychometric system.' *Medical and Biological Engineering,* 10, 145.
Brown, C. C., Whitman, J. R. (1963) 'Apparatus for measuring restricted ranges of linear movement.' *American Journal of Psychology,* 76, 138.
Challacombe, D. N., MacCulloch, M. J., Birtles, C. J. (1972) 'Controlled measures of exploratory movement in a coeliac child during gluten withdrawal.' *Archive of Diseases in Childhood,* 47, 823.
Chess, S. (1960) 'Diagnosis and treatment of the hyperactive child.' *New York State Journal of Medicine,* 60, 2379.
Currie, K. H., Brannigan, C. R. (1968) 'Behavioural analysis and modification with an autistic child.' *In* Hutt, S. J., Hutt, C. (Eds.) *Behaviour Studies in Psychiatry.* Oxford and New York: Pergamon Press, pp. 77-90.
Grant, E. C. (1968) Personal communication.
Grant, Q. R. (1962) 'Psychopharmacology in childhood emotional and mental disorders.' *Journal of Pediatrics,* 61, 626.
Kenny, T. J., Clemmens, R. L., Hudson, B. W., Lentz, G. A., Cicci, R., Nair, P. (1971) 'Characteristics of children referred because of hyperactivity.' *Journal of Pediatrics,* 79, 618.
Ko, W. H., Neuman, M. R. (1967) 'Implant biotelemetry and microelectronics.' *Science,* 156, 351.

Longo, N., Pellegrino, J. W. (1967) 'A simple telemetric method for monitoring cardiac function in small animals.' *Perceptual and Motor Skills,* **24,** 512.

MacCulloch, M. J., Birtles, C. J., Bond, S. (1969) 'A free space-time traversal data-logging system for two human subjects.' *Medical and Biological Engineering,* **7,** 593.

—— Williams, C., Davies, P. (1971) 'Heart rate variability in a group of cerebral palsied children.' *Developmental Medicine and Child Neurology,* **13,** 645.

—— Williams, C. (1971) 'On the nature of infantile autism.' *Acta Psychiatrica Scandinavica,* **47,** 295.

Mitchell, S., Shepherd, M. (1966) 'A comparative study of children's behaviour at home and at school.' *British Journal of Educational Psychology,* **36,** 248.

Moore, R., Goldiamond, I. (1964) 'Errorless establishment of visual discrimination using fading procedures.' *Journal of the Experimental Analysis of Behaviour,* **7,** 269.

Ounsted, C. (1955) 'The hyperkinetic syndrome in epileptic children.' *Lancet,* **ii,** 303.

Patterson, G. R., Jones, R., Whittier, J., Wright, M. A. (1971) 'A behaviour modification technique for the hyperactive child.' *In* Graziano, A. M. (Ed.) *Behavior Therapy with Children.* Chicago: Aldine-Atherton.

Rutter, M., Graham, P. (1966) 'Psychiatric disorder in ten and eleven year old children.' *Proceedings of the Royal Society of Medicine,* **59,** 382.

—— Tizard, J., Whitmore, K. (1972) *Education, Health and Behaviour.* London: Longman, pp. 147-177.

Sambrooks, J. E., MacCulloch, M. J., Birtles, C. J., Smallman, C. (1972) 'Assessment of the effects of flurazepam and nitrazepam on visuo-motor performance using an automated assessment technique.' *Acta Psychiatrica Scandinavica,* **48,** 443.

Stattleman, A., Cook, H. (1966) 'A transducer for motion study by radio telemetry.' *Proceedings of the Society for Experimental Biology and Medicine,* **121,** 505.

Stewart, M. A., Pitts, F. N., Craig, A. G., Dierfu, W. (1966) 'The hyperactive child syndrome.' *American Journal of Ortho-Psychiatry,* **35,** 861.

Ullmann, C. A. (1952) *Identification of Maladjusted School Children.* U.S. Public Health Monograph. No. 7.

Underwood Committee (1955) *Report of the Committee on Maladjusted Children.* London: H.M.S.O.

Weiss, A. L. (1929) 'The measurement of infant behaviour.' *Psychological Review,* **36,** 453.

Werry, J. S., Weiss, G., Douglas, V., Martin, J. (1968) 'Studies on the hyperactive child: the effect of chlorpromazine on behaviour and learning ability.' *In* Quay, H. (Ed.) *Children's Behavior Disorders: an Enduring Problem in Psychology.* New York: Van Nostrand.

THERAPEUTIC AND EDUCATIONAL
APPLICATIONS

A Developmental Intervention Programme Designed to Overcome the Effects of Impaired Movement in Spina Bifida Infants

P. ROSENBAUM, R. BARNITT and H. LORNA BRAND

The work described here is one of the variations on a theme, *viz.* the relationship between mobility and early learning, which Dr. Holt and several of his colleagues at The Wolfson Centre have been studying for some time. More precisely, we have pondered the effects of early and prolonged impairment of mobility on the development of young children. Our study grew out of earlier observations by Rosenbloom and Horton of hand function in non-disabled children and in children with spina bifida. They noted clumsy hand use in both gross and fine motor tasks in the children with spina bifida. It was also noted that these children needed to use their arms and hands to assist their mobility, suggesting that perhaps part of the impairment of function might have resulted from a lack of opportunity to use their hands in play as do ordinary children. Rosenbloom and Horton also found that a programme of activities aimed at training hand function led to improvements in dexterity and a lessening of clumsiness (Rosenbloom and Horton, 1972, *personal communication*).

It seemed appropriate, therefore, to look at a larger group of young children with spina bifida and try to prevent those deficits of upper limb function that were found in the older children.

Several factors influenced the decision to select children with spina bifida for our study: the condition is detectable at birth; such infants are likely to have early and prolonged impairment of mobility; compared with a population of, say, cerebral palsied children, the children with spina bifida form a relatively more homogenous group; and the prevalence of spina bifida in the south of England is such that an adequate study population was available.

Finally, an important consideration was the fact that a longitudinal study of the development of such children was already being carried out by Miss Bernie Spain, a research psychologist working under the aegis of the Greater London Council (Spain 1970). Miss Spain had begun to characterise the developmental patterns of about 170 children. Of particular interest was her finding of a tendency, detectable at one year of age and obvious by three years, for relatively poor development of hand-eye co-ordination compared with language or personal/social development. This tended to confirm the observations of Rosenbloom and Horton, and to imply that factors occurring very early in life were contributing to impaired hand function. It is relevant to add that Miss Spain's data provided base-line observations against which we would eventually measure our study population. We were able to compare our group with that part of her group treated at the same hospital some three to five years earlier by the same staff and in a relatively similar fashion.

The intervention programme was based upon our personal experiences and reviews of relevant literature. We were aware, from both sources, that most parents of young handicapped children need a great deal of emotional and practical support in raising such children. To cite briefly two studies: Shere and Kastenbaum (1966) clearly highlighted the fact that parents and specialists concerned with cerebral palsied children usually failed to appreciate the effects of physical disability upon cognitive growth and development, and 'as a result, the children were raised in an almost barren environment, which prevented them from gaining experience of the object world'. Similarly, Larson's (1958) work indicated that physically handicapped children had significant deficits in their early experiences compared with ordinary controls. These deficits were evident not only in physical activities such as hiking in the woods or going to the shops, but were equally marked in areas of knowledge and experience, such as knowing the story 'Goldilocks and the Three Bears'.

In planning our study, we therefore attempted to help the parents understand and appreciate the effects of motor impairment upon other non-physical aspects of development. We wished to study the developmental achievements of the children and offer advice appropriate to the stages of development reached at each age. In this aspect of the study we were helped considerably by the work of Dr. Reynell, who outlined four principles to be considered in planning treatment programmes for pre-school handicapped children (Reynell 1973).

(1) *Developmental orientation*
An approach based on a clear understanding of the principles and patterns of normal child development; an assessment of the present developmental achievements of a handicapped child; and a programme designed to build upon current abilities in a developmentally appropriate sequence.

(2) *Flexibility*
A suitable programme must take account of the individuality and variations among children inherent even within a group of children with apparently similar disabilities.

(3) *Simple equipment*
With young children being cared for at home or in nurseries, it is important that any toys or materials required be inexpensive and readily available.

(4) *Simple programme*
If the model is to be widely applicable, it must be easy to carry out, even partly by parents in the home.

Lastly, we wished to observe the emergence of hand-eye co-ordinated skills. Although other aspects of development were not ignored, a programme of specific activities was developed which emphasised the training of hand-eye co-ordination. The programme was designed so that it could be carried out by the parents in their hour to hour and day to day handling of their infants.

Intervention Programme

The practical advice given to the parents was based on the following plan.

0 TO 3 MONTHS

1.   VISUAL FIXATION expected to emerge and to develop significantly in first month.

TRAINING
   (a)   The mother should look at the baby and smile and coo while feeding. The babies often stare at the mother during feeding.
   (b)   The baby is shown the bottle; visual fixation is rewarded with immediate feeding.

2.   VISUAL FOLLOWING seen in second month. Horizontal following precedes vertical.

TRAINING
   (a)   When fixation is well established (see 1b) visual following (not fixation) is rewarded. Same sequence of events is carried a step further; slow, deliberate movements of objects with gradual increase in range of movement. When horizontal following is well established, vertical movement is introduced.
   (b)   The same thing can be done with the infant following the mother's face. Visual following is rewarded with smiling, cooing and cuddling.

3.   GRASPING AN OBJECT PLACED IN THE HANDS should occur in latter part of third month. Voluntary grasp and brief holding of an object are to be expected. (This is *not* a reflex at this stage.)

TRAINING
   (a)   When the baby is relaxed and happy, with hands open, an object such as a wooden rod or ring is placed in his hands. The mother then plays at removing it, pulling the object and hand about playfully.

3 TO 6 MONTHS

4.   GRASP AND PLAY WITH OBJECTS follows from *3* above. It evolves gradually and can be trained easily.

TRAINING
   (a)   The baby is shown an attractive or favourite toy; as soon as visual fixation and interest are noted, the object is put in the baby's hand.
   (b)   The mother plays at removing the object.
   (c)   One now expects to see a sensorimotor link, *i.e.* the child begins to open its hands in anticipation of the object. The child is rewarded with the object only when these efforts are made.

(d)   More and more active effort is expected from the baby. Arm movements towards the object are rewarded in a graded way as performance improves.

5.   REACH AND GRASP follow logically.

TRAINING
(a)   When the level of achievement of *4d* is well established, the baby's range of reaching should be extended. This is done by offering favourite toys from various positions in front of and to each side of the baby. The reward is the toy, reinforced by maternal praise.

6.   MOUTHING is usually seen around the age of 20 to 24 weeks.

TRAINING
(a)   The mother is encouraged to allow the baby to feed himself. When mouthing begins, it can usually be reinforced by giving the baby dry rusks as these are intrinsically rewarding.
(b)   Reaching and holding behaviours are reinforced with feeding. Babies at this age often bring both hands up to hold the bottle.

6 TO 9 MONTHS

7.   UNIDEXTROUS APPROACH should appear from about the seventh month onwards.

TRAINING
(a)   This should be done with the baby well supported in sitting position at a table or good surface. Attractive or noise-making toys are offered from many positions which require unilateral reaching.
(b)   The baby should also learn to secure objects from a surface, *e.g.* table or bench. This is encouraged by the parent taking the baby's hand, placing it on the object, and picking it up with him.

8.   TRANSFER OF OBJECTS FROM HAND TO HAND is encouraged around the seventh month.

TRAINING
(a)   A toy is offered from one side of the baby. When the baby has secured the toy, both his hands are brought together onto the toy and the baby is helped to transfer the toy from one hand to the other. This is done from both sides. Successful behaviour is rewarded with praise.

9.   TWO OBJECTS RETAINED SIMULTANEOUSLY

TRAINING
(a)   Two similar objects are offered one after the other to the baby. Success is

rewarded with play and praise.
(b) Two pieces of favourite food may be offered.

10. OBJECT PERMANENCE is first seen in terms of looking after a fallen object. This develops into an ablility to remember where an object has gone when it is seen to disappear.

TRAINING
(a) A favourite object is deliberately knocked from the table. The baby is asked where it has gone, and it is then produced immediately by the parent. This is done several times in succession. Gradually, the duration of absence from view is increased to several seconds. At first, any reaching behaviour is rewarded, but later, only the more relevant searching movements are rewarded.
(b) When the baby has grasped the idea of looking and searching for objects in this way, the parent plays games of covering an object, first only partially (with hand or cloth) then totally. Motor behaviour aimed at reaching the toy is rewarded with praise and, of course, with the toy itself.

9 TO 12 MONTHS

11. THE PINCER GRASP is used from about the age of nine months, with gradually increasing sophistication.

TRAINING
(a) Finger feeding is perhaps the best way to encourage this. Bite-sized pieces of food are offered one at a time and are given only in response to pincer-like movement. As the pincer grasp improves, smaller pieces of food are offered.

12. THE INDEX APPROACH is seen at about ten months of age.

TRAINING
(a) The baby is encouraged to imitate his parent, by pointing at objects.
(b) The parent makes a game of poking an index finger through an opening, e.g. in an empty tissue box, to secure a sweet. The child imitates the parent.

13. RELEASE OF OBJECTS begins at about the eleventh month.

TRAINING
(a) The parent plays at 'give and take', offering toys to the baby and expecting them back.
(b) The baby is encouraged to pick up objects such as small wooden bricks, and release them into a container such as a metal pot. The rewards are the various noises made by the bricks hitting the pot.

149

The babies in this project were admitted to our hospital from local maternity hospitals. This meant that they were separated from their mothers for the first few days of life. This separation, plus the fact the babies were handicapped, resulted in many of the mothers being nervous of handling their children less efficiently than the nurses. On the whole, therefore, they were pleased to be involved in a practical programme which would help their babies' development. Not all the fathers were co-operative initially; they were concerned about what was being done to their children.

The family was introduced to the first stage of the programme at the first out-patient visit, when the baby was four to six weeks old. As babies of this age sleep a great deal, the first part of the programme centred around feeding times, when they are at their most alert. The mother was encouraged to interact as much as possible with the baby, and more specifically, was asked to show the bottle to the baby before feeding, and reward visual fixation by giving the feed. In the early stages, it was often doubtful whether the baby had looked at the bottle or not; he was, however, usually given the benefit of the doubt at this stage. The situation was intended to be pleasant and rewarding, and not one which brought any stress into the mother/baby relationship.

Although the procedure may sound very simple, several mothers said that they had not realised that this response was possible in such young babies, and with their older children, had simply pushed the bottle into the baby's mouth. The families therefore became aware from a very early stage that they had a child to interact with and not just a passive baby who needed caring for.

Once the baby had learnt to fix his gaze on the bottle and then on his mother's face, the mother was told to bring her face close to the child and slowly move her face in a horizontal plane. The baby was always rewarded for following successfully. (Throughout the project, stress was placed on adequate reward to reinforce the desired behaviour.) At this particular stage, reward consisted of smiling, cuddling and verbal stimulation from the mother or father.

During early clinic visits, the babies were accompanied by both parents whenever possible, and both parents were encouraged to become involved in the programme.

Towards the end of the first three months the development of hand skills was stimulated by placing small objects in the babies' open hands.

During the second three months of life the baby learns that he does not have to rely on his parents to initiate his movements. He learns that he can use his hands to reach out and gain objects. The parents initiated this activity by showing the baby a toy, and, when the baby looked at it, placing this toy in the baby's hands. We always demonstrated to the parents the degree of visual fixation and interest which we expected from the child before he was rewarded. We also emphasised the importance of rewarding the child immediately he was successful, so that he could associate looking at the object with his receiving it. The child must be interested in the game and show pleasure in achieving the object if he is going to benefit from the programme.

From the sixth month onwards, those children who had not achieved independent sitting were placed in chairs on the floor. In this way the children were able to emulate the activities encountered by normal children sitting independently. If the child is placed on the floor without a chair, he must use his hands to support himself, and therefore has no chance to develop hand skills. Also, the handicap child sitting in a high chair cannot watch objects move away from, towards and around him.

When the child was between six and 12 months old, the parents received demonstrations and advice on the early stages of mobility. They were shown, for instance, how to initiate rolling behaviour by turning the baby's head to look for a toy. We found that unless instructions were demonstrated, they were often interpreted in a wide variety of ways. For example, when helping the baby to pick up bricks and put them in a container, the containers chosen were often far too shallow. This meant that the babies did not have a clear idea of the action of 'putting in' and 'taking out'. Conversely, the containers were sometimes so deep that the child could not see where the brick was going.

In addition to these specific activities, the parents were encouraged to give their children crayons, paper, paints and to introduce various kinds of free play appropriate to the level of motor achievement reached by the child. Children who had not developed any mobility were placed near cupboards or given cardboard boxes of toys to empty, in order to encourage the parents to help in providing normal play situations.

When the children had become accustomed to sitting on the floor with their hands free for play, the physiotherapist then supplied 'standers'. The 'standers' enabled the child to see the world from an upright position and to play in an upright position with his hands quite free. They were not designed to serve primarily as aids to mobility and walking. Throughout the programme, no stress was laid on the achievement of skills by any definite chronological age, as we did not want the parents to be unduly anxious about their children's development. Most of the families knew, and, over a period of time, were able to accept that the handicapped baby was not as bright as their other children.

Organisation of the Study

The study was carried out at the Queen Elizabeth Hospital, London, by a team consisting of a physiotherapist, occupational therapist and paediatrician. The occupational therapist (as a full-time member of the hospital staff) provided many of the vital links between the research and primary care aspects of patient management, and gave advice to the families between research visits and after completion of the study programme.

The study group consisted of all babies with spina bifida admitted to the care of one paediatric surgeon between September 1971 and June 1972 and to a second surgeon between April and June 1972. The 19 infants (11 males, eight females) who survived the neonatal period were included in the study. Fourteen infants had Spitz-Holter valves for the control of hydrocephalus.

The general pattern of assessments is shown in Table I. At two to four weeks, following surgery to the back and usually insertion of a valve, the babies were seen on the ward for an initial paediatric and neurodevelopmental evaluation. This first assessment was particularly useful in providing information about the probable degree of neurological impairment. We met the parents at the initial out-patient visit, usually when the babies were four to six weeks old. The surgeon introduced us to the parents as 'professionals with an interest in the development of your child', and we explained that we would like the opportunity to watch the baby grow and develop. We also told the parents that we could offer ideas for play and management which we hoped would foster the child's development.

Developmental assessments were carried out at three, six and 12 months of age. Many of these later assessments were carried out at the children's homes. At these visits we discussed appropriate aspects of the hand-eye stimulation programme, demonstrating the child's current abilities and showing the parents how present motor achievements could be expected to change and develop in the ensuing weeks.

The therapists made a point of knowing in advance about any visit of a study infant to the hospital, in order to see the infant and to chat with the parents. By so doing they were able to reinforce advice offered at the more formal training sessions, and to answer any questions the parents might have. This meant that the programme of visuomotor training was taught and demonstrated more frequently than is implied by the schedule of visits shown in Table I.

TABLE I

Pattern of assessments

Age	Place	Procedure
2 to 4 weeks	Hospital ward	Neurodevelopmental paediatric assessment
4 to 6 weeks	Clinic	Meet parents, introduction and discussion
3 months	Clinic	Developmental assessment and programme
6 months	Clinic or home	Developmental assessment and programme
12 months	Clinic or home	Developmental assessment, Griffiths scales and developmental evaluation

By ten to 14 months of age many babies were attending regular fortnightly mobility sessions, and it then became possible to increase the visuomotor training programme considerably.

On or soon after their first birthday, all babies were independently assessed by Miss Bernie Spain, using the Griffiths Developmental Scales to evaluate locomotor, personal/social, language, hand-eye, and performance abilities of the children.

Results

Of the 19 infants in the study, one died at eight months, another was not available at the time of assessment, and a third was severely mentally retarded. The omission of these children accounts for the varying numbers in the tables.

At six months of age, six infants sat appropriately for their age, five could sit momentarily but did not have their hands free, and eight infants had no useful trunk control even when supported.

At twelve months of age, eight infants could sit independently and had full freedom of hand use, while nine were considered abnormal because their hands were still partly or completely required for support.

In considering the locomotor abilities, we divided our observations into two parts, recording both what the child was able to do and what he actually did do. (See Table II.) It is interesting to note that, where locomotor abilities are fairly age-appropriately developed, they are used, but with the more severely handicapped children, lack of motivation seems at least as important as impaired gross motor function. Almost half the children hardly moved at all, although four of these could roll. The one infant who did use rolling was actively exploring his environment and taking full advantage of this ability.

TABLE II
Locomotor abilities of 17 infants at 12 months

Locomotor ability	Can do	Does do
Walk unaided	2	2
Walk with aid	3	3
Creep/crawl/pivot	3	3
Roll	5	I
No Movement	4	8
Total	17	17

Neurodevelopmental evaluation of upper limb function was carried out at one year of age. Subtle evidence of abnormality was suggested by the findings of mild to moderate asymmetry of hand preference in seven infants. In several instances there was also evidence of posturing of the hands, mild decrease in tone and strength of upper limbs, or decreased range of movement at the shoulders. One infant had a dense left hemiplegia acquired at nine months of age, while another showed diminished power and tone of both arms without evident impairment of function. Two infants were developmentally very immature without localised neurological deficits, and seven showed no neurodevelopmental problems in their upper limbs.

Visual assessment at one year revealed one child with a squint and left hemianopia, and one with a squint and suspected decreased acuity possibly coupled with impaired visual fields.

Assessment of the success of the intervention programme was based primarily on developmental evaluation as measured by the Griffiths Scales. The results are given in Tables VIII. Group 1 refers to the 30 children in Miss Spain's study who were treated at the Queen Elizabeth Hospital during the period April 1967 to March 1969. This group is used as the reference group against which our study group (Group 2) has been compared.

The letters in the tables refer to the areas evaluated in the Griffiths tests, as follows: A, locomotor; B, personal, social; C, hearing, speech; D, hand-eye co-ordination; and E, performance ability.

Considering all the children (Table III), there appears to be little difference between the two groups. Because Miss Spain had found that a locomotor score at one year of age of 60 or more seemed predictive of later aided or unaided walking, we divided the groups up in this way for further analysis.

153

In the groups with locomotor scores of 60 or higher (Table IV), the study population seemed slightly above the average in all spheres of development, and scored higher than the other group throughout. However, if the gross motor score (column A) is any indication of severity of lesion, then the study group was significantly less disabled than the earlier group. Concerning the groups with locomotor scores of 60 or less (Table V) the reverse would seem to be true, with the study group (Group 2) performing slightly less well throughout.

A further analysis of the results was made in the following way. As the D and E scales of the Griffiths test both measure (directly or indirectly) aspects of hand-eye behaviour, these scores were combined. Similarly, the scores on the B and C scales, both measuring abilities reflecting social development, were also combined.

In both Table VII and Table VIII the Group I totals for B plus C and D plus E are about equal or are unremarkably different, whereas in Group 2 the totals for D plus E are respectively nine and ten points higher than the B plus C totals. Thus within Group 2 there is a tendency towards better performance in visuomotor tasks (*i.e.* those towards which the training programme was directed) compared with aspects of development that were not trained. Furthermore, these results suggest that it is possible, with appropriate intervention advice and activities, to reverse the trend toward relatively poor hand-eye co-ordination in these children. These results apply regardless of the severity of the motor impairment.

TABLE III
Mean Griffiths scores of all children

	No. of children	(With valves)	A	B	C	D	E
Group 1	30	11	69	101	104	99	104
Group 2	16	11	72	97	98	101	104

TABLE IV
Mean Griffiths scores of children with locomotor score > 60

	No. of children	(With valves)	A	B	C	D	E
Group 1	18	9	79	104	106	102	109
Group 2	7	3	102	109	108	111	115

TABLE V
Mean Griffiths scores of children with locomotor score < 60

	No. of children	(With valves)	A	B	C	D	E
Group 1	12	10	52	96	100	95	98
Group 2	9	8	45	87	90	93	94

TABLE VI
Mean Griffiths scores of all children

	No. of children	A	B and C	D and E
Group 1	30	69	205	203
Group 2	16	72	195	205

TABLE VII
Mean Griffiths scores of children with locomotor score > 60

	No. of children	A	B and C	D and E
Group 1	18	79	210	211
Group 2	7	102	217	226

TABLE VIII
Mean Griffiths scores of children with locomotor score < 60

	No. of children	A	B and C	D and E
Group 1	12	52	196	193
Group 2	9	45	177	187

Discussion

Although not very dramatic, the results do tend to support the original hypothesis and the value of the intervention programme. That the results were not more striking is probably due to the multiple etiology of the problem. It is almost certainly true that any specific disability found in children with spina bifida will be multi-determined. For example, most children with spina bifida have some degree of hydrocephalus; many children have minor degrees of neurological impairment of their upper limbs; there are known to be perceptual difficulties in older youngsters; children with spina bifida have prolonged and repeated hospital admissions and their families experience a high incidence of social upheaval and emotional stress. The impaired mobility is thus seen as only one of several possible influences on development.

Unfortunately, we did not look in detail at the social or attitudinal factors in the study families, nor did we measure any of these factors. Our impression was that much of the value of the programme lay in the general factors which were part of the design of the study e.g. unlimited time, general as well as specific developmental advice, and an interest in the parents as well as their infants. We had little doubt, from the comments of parents and hospital staff, that the babies were being reared with greater confidence and satisfaction than previously.

REFERENCES

Larson, L. (1958) 'Preschool experiences of physically handicapped children.' *Exceptional Children,* **74,** 310.

Reynell, J. K. (1973) 'Planning treatment programmes: pre-school children.' *In* Mittler, P. (Ed.) *Assessment for Learning in the Mentally Handicapped.* Edinburgh and London: Churchill Livingstone.

Shere, E., Kastenbaum, R. (1966) 'Mother-child interaction in cerebral palsy: environmental and psycho-social obstacles to cognitive development.' *Genetic Psychology Monographs,* **73,** 255.

Spain, B. (1970) 'Spina bifida survey.' *Greater London Council Intelligence Unit. Quarterly Bulletin,* no. 12, 5.

CHAPTER FOURTEEN

The Rôle of Music in the Stimulation of Movement

PRISCILLA BARCLAY

'Since music be so good a thing,
I wish all men would learn to sing.'
An old Round

Throughout the ages music has been an immensely important influence. It has been described as the most civilising of the arts, and indeed, Plato insisted that music should be included in the education of young Greeks.

Music has a great influence on behaviour and can affect the quality of people's responses to their environment. It reaches the body, mind and spirit, bringing to a discouraging environment a quality and beauty hitherto absent.

Therefore, when we talk of music stimulating *movement*, we include the bodily, mental and spiritual reactions (of the child) to music. Sometimes a reaction is manifest only in the eyes, or by a smile, or sometimes the child may lift his head so that his lips touch a pipe or recorder played close to him. This movement of reaching to the instrument may spread through the whole body lying in bed, with the result that the child has moved, has experienced movement, and something has stirred in him.

When a child cannot use speech to express himself, he uses his body. His movements, gestures and actions, become his language. The violence of his actions and the turbulence of his behaviour show his distress and are his cry for help.

In addition to initiating movement, music can also guide and control action, and interpret emotion. In order to be of benefit in bringing about development and growth towards a more harmonious and satisfactory way of life for the child, the use of music must be practical and within the understanding of the child.

At St. Lawrence's*, Caterham, the use of music is adapted to suit the needs of the individual. The children have individual sessions and/or work in small groups, where the work is adapted to the extent of their mobility.

The Way in which Music is Used

Almost all children *react* to music. This reaction may be great or small, but it indicates that sound (in this case, musical sound) has impinged upon the child's consciousness. This is the first step.

Next comes a *conscious response,* an urge towards the sound that has given pleasure and a desire to have the sound repeated. This is the second step.

The third step is the child's own effort to create the sound, leading to *creative*

---

*St. Lawrence's, Caterham, Surrey, is a hospital for the severely subnormal, where many of the children have multiple handicaps and other ills in addition to their mental retardation.

achievement. This may involve being one of a group making music, or playing an instrument really well.

We have, thus, three levels of response from a child, *viz.*, *reaction*, *conscious response* and *creative achievement*.

Three basic elements of music are used:
(1) tempo (fast/slow);
(2) dynamics (loud/soft);
(3) form (realisation of tempo and dynamics within a given framework).

The first thing needed in any music session is an attitude of listening. To obtain this the children are given coloured hoops, large coloured balls and musical notes made from fairly large pieces of plywood. These serve as a focus for attention and concentration. Also, the children prefer to make these toys do what the music says than listen to verbal instructions from an adult.

Each child has a ball and when the music is played in treble he throws it in the air and catches it again; when the music is changed to bass, the ball is bounced on the floor and caught again. For those with good co-ordination and control, the throwing, catching and bouncing can be done simultaneously while walking, running or skipping.

Having got the children into a state of listening and alertness, the first basic element is now introduced.

Tempo

The music does not keep to the same speed all the time, it goes faster or slower. The children each choose a plywood symbol and as the music plays at the speed of walking (♩), running (♫), and slow (𝅗𝅥), the child (or children) who holds the appropriate symbol moves about the room at the speed indicated. The music changes frequently from one speed to another, and no-one may move until the speed corresponding to his symbol is played, and he may only continue his action of walking or running while the music is playing at that speed. Two or three note values are then played at the same time, so that the children are moving about at different speeds. This leads to a member of the group taking over the rôle of pace-setter from the pianist. One child becomes the conductor and makes the groups of notes move as he wants. This calls for a degree of leadership, as the child who leads must dominate his companions and get them all following his wishes; he must know what he wants and must make his own decisions.

There are many ways of using the notes, all calling for controlled movement, co-ordination and aural discrimination. The notes, for example, may be laid on the floor to form a rhythmic pattern as in ♩ ♩ ♫ ♩ ♫/𝅗𝅥 𝅗𝅥// (walk walk run run slow slow). This pattern is clapped and spoken in words descriptive of action, and then it is stepped and perhaps analysed so that a child can write it on the blackboard. The fact that a child is able to step such a rhythm means that a fine control of movement has been achieved.

Dynamics

In musical terms, dynamic changes consist of the following: forte/piano

158

(loud/soft); crescendo/diminuendo (getting louder/getting softer); staccato/legato (jumpy, abrupt playing/smooth playing); different harmonies; concords and discords; and the effect of different intervals.

In the early stages, these changes in the dynamics of the music are best introduced to the children while they are seated on the floor, as this gives them a feeling of security and also removes any problems of balance. Each child has a coloured ball, which he moves in imitation of the music. For example, he shows 'staccato' by a sharp movement of hand and wrist which makes the ball spin. By using the tune of 'Twinkle, Twinkle, Little Star', various gradations of muscular energy are called forth by playing the music loudly and energetically (the child is told that the star is glittering energetically and so must spin the ball fiercely), or softly (the child spins the ball gently). This exercise involves movements which are concentrated and close to the body.

By taking another tune, such as 'I Saw Three Ships Come Sailing By', the action of rolling a ball along the floor is suggested. The musician again governs the quality of the rollings by the loudness or softness of his playing. The physical movement involved here is now a flowing movement away from the body.

Subtle changes in the child's feelings towards the music may be brought about by changing key and harmonies from concord to discord. A very musical child may be quite startled by the changes and want to know what has been done to the tune.

All these changes of dynamics are followed instantaneously by the children and there is real communication between them and the player as movements become freer and responses more sensitive.

Form

The third element of music *studied* is form (design or pattern). The word 'studied' is used here because a more intellectual effort is required from the children than with tempo or dynamics.

The material used is the sequence of phrases and simple construction of a folk tune, *e.g.* 'Pop Goes the Weasel'. A sequence of four or eight phrases forms the framework upon which a movement design is constructed. Again, the scheme is very simple. The beginning of the tune has a skipping rhythm and ends with the exclamation 'Pop goes the weasel', which is very distinct and easy to hear. Thus, starting from within a coloured hoop placed on the floor, the children skip around and away from the hoop quite freely at the beginning of the tune. Then the words 'Pop goes the weasel' are changed to 'Jump in the hoop' at which command each child must jump back into his coloured hoop. The children quickly learn the distance they may travel during the skipping period in order to be able to return to the hoop in good time for the final phrase—not too soon and not in a mad rush from the other side of the room. From the point of view of distance covered, limits are set beyond which the child may not go.

Subsequently, the children acquire a feeling for the length or measure of a phrase. Each phrase ends with a cadence, and the feeling for and recognition of this cadence is demonstrated by the children in the following way: carrying their hoops they move freely during the course of a phrase and at the cadence (end of musical phrase) they touch another person's hoop with their own. In this way the child also becomes aware of his companions, as he must keep an eye open to be sure that he is near enough to someone else to touch hoops at the end of the phrase.

When the feeling for phrase is established, the phrases of the melody can be built into a design. This is done by ascribing each phrase of the tune to a particular child. If there are four phrases, four children (carrying their hoops) place themselves in various positions around the room. The first child's name is called and he goes off to a spot chosen by himself. As the second, third and fourth phrases are played the names of the second, third and fourth children are called and they must then go off and touch hoops with the first child. This can also be done by calling the colours of the hoops instead of names. Some children may stretch out to touch, others may kneel; each child may take any position he likes that enables him to touch the hoop of the first. Each child has freedom of choice within this given framework, the limits of which must be respected.

From this basic training of learning to move to what he has heard and discovered in the music, many other prospects open up for the child.

Stories in Music

Stories in music help to draw together all that has been absorbed previously. A simple nativity play performed to the carol of 'The Friendly Beasts' (based on the phrasing work) and 'Joshua Fit de Battle of Jericho' (based on the conducting work) gave a group of St. Lawrence's boys both great joy and pride and brought out a sense of responsibility that was remarkable.

The children acquire a simple vocabulary which can be used in endless ways to stimulate imagination and spontaneity of movement. The construction of the music, its tempo and rhythm, dynamics, harmony and form, not only stimulate movement, but become familiar material with which the children can stimulate themselves and so actively and consciously further their own development. Perhaps most important of all is the great enjoyment they take in these activities, for it is on this enjoyment that the effectiveness of the work depends. The therapist and children must share the musical experience and interaction between them must be happy and lively as both take pleasure in the music.

The Therapist

What is the therapist's rôle in all this? How does the therapist help the child imprisoned by his disabilities to achieve greater freedom of movement and become a more harmonious and happier person? First, she must have empathy with the child, must feel with him and, through music, speak to him. She needs training in movement in order to feel and express outwardly the movement in the music. Her bodily attitude, voice and gestures must be sensitive and expressive if she is to develop feeling and sensitivity to the music and bring this to the awareness of the child. A wide knowledge and training is essential, she must think through music and, like a painter choosing his colours, must be able to combine and contrast the different elements of music.

As it is difficult to find exactly what one requires in various musical compositions, the therapist must often improvise the composition to suit her purpose. Few therapists are great composers, just as few people speak in great poetry, but the therapist must at least be able to speak simply and grammatically in music. She must be able to produce music which will elicit the desired responses from the patients, and also adapt the music to fit the needs and impulses of the patients at any given moment. For example, if the child stops moving sooner than expected, then an ordinary four-bar phrase should be curtailed to a three-bar phrase. Likewise, if the child moves for longer than expected, four bars must be extended into five. The same rule applies to sudden, unpredictable changes of mood; these must be followed by a corresponding change in the music so that immediate and constant contact is made and maintained.

Composed music, from record or tape, or played by the therapist, also has its place in therapy. The children respond to fine music either by intense listening or by moving themselves spontaneously to it. This listening also creates a group feeling and children who do not perhaps take much notice of each other become united in the act of listening together.

Every therapy session should have a session of quiet listening, during which the children can relax and concentrate on the music. Continual, loud background music from radio or television simply numbs the children and damages the close interaction between the children and therapist.

Children in Wheel-chairs

What has been described has been the work done with mobile children of low intelligence, but music can also give the same pleasure and sense of achievement to children confined to wheel-chairs.

Musical instruments can be adapted to suit the individual child. For example, a cymbal can be played with a specially-designed beater, and this and other instruments can provide good musical accompaniment to a melody played on the pipe, flute, violin or piano. Songs, too, can be effectively accompanied in this way.

Speech Difficulties

Children with speech difficulties can often be helped through singing. The movements for speech can be practised and are often initiated in this way.

Assessment

Assessment of success or failure in music therapy cannot really be measured by ordinary standards. Many things have to be considered, such as the child's physical age and condition, his intelligence, his treatment prior to music therapy, his past/present everyday environment, *etc.*

Ideally, treatment and everyday life should be one continuous process, the result of team work carried out consistently by all concerned with the child, with each specialist contributing to the total developmental progress.

CHAPTER FIFTEEN

The Rôle of Physical Education in the Stimulation of Movement

A. BROWN

Physical Education is concerned with movement and the benefits which accrue from the improved quality of movement. These benefits include increased *skill*, greater *physical fitness*, better *social development* and greater *enjoyment* of leisure.

During the early years of a handicapped child's life, the people most concerned with his physical education are his parents and physiotherapists. Later, the Physical Education teacher attempts to encourage abilities within the limited movement potential of the child. This can lead to the development of sub-skills and eventually to skills which enable the child to participate in various activities of physical recreation.

My experience comes from teaching cerebral palsied children of normal intelligence. For an energetic and imaginative teacher, mildly disabled children are no different from normal children. The greatest problem is the difficulty of stimulating gross movement patterns in severely handicapped quadriplegic, athetoid and ataxic children, especially where previous attempts at skilful movement have failed, or where such movements may not even be possible because of severe perceptuo-motor problems. Where movement is limited and of a low order, the most significant difficulty facing the teacher is *motivation*. Both in physical education and daily living, the highest motivating force in stimulating prolonged practice is success. It is also necessary to establish, in the mind of the learner, the *need* for practice, while at the same time holding out a realistic *hope of success*. *The teacher, therefore, must help the handicapped child to be successful and to gain satisfaction from seeing discernible progress in the acquisition of skill.*

The teacher must institute a progressive scheme of learning so that simple goals are achieved steadily and motivation remains high. Also, suitable skills and the adaptation of these skills in performance must be carefully selected. It is most important that the skill chosen is valued in the eyes of the learner; it should not be a puerile activity such as dropping pennies into a bucket. Selection of material is critical when dealing with teenage girls and here, perhaps, the aesthetic aspects of Physical Education should be given greater emphasis, *e.g.* dance, music and movement, drama, *etc.*

It is useful to consider those skills that a severely handicapped child can perform on a personal, individual basis and those that he can perform as part of a group. In the first case, a successful performance often shows considerable improvement. However, in the case of group activities, the teacher must be careful to ensure that the child has a definite rôle to play and is not present merely in body. The child who senses he is not contributing may feel a failure, and, in this way, psychological damage can occur.

Without a basic level of ability in certain skills (throwing a ball, catching it, stopping it) a child is necessarily excluded from team games. To enable the child to achieve these skills, the teacher must analyse the perceptuo-motor problems of each child and integrate these into a programme of *progressive development and adaptation.*

Progressive Development and Adaptation: an Example

In order to carry out the simple action of catching a ball, the player watches its flight, perceives its speed, height, spin and direction; on the basis of experience he then predicts where it is likely to fall and makes a decision as to when and where to position his hands. Failure to catch the ball may be due to an error at any stage of the performance; for example, poor tracking of flight, error in hand placement, failure to close grasp at the right moment, commencing effector response too late, *etc.* By analysing this simple task one can appreciate how complex it must be for the severely handicapped child with visuo-motor and perceptuo-motor difficulties. In order to teach the child, one must first simplify the task. This may be done in the following way.

(1) When a ball is rolled along the ground, the path of the ball becomes two-dimensional (in terms of speed and direction) and its future position is easier to predict than if it were thrown in the air. It also helps if the ball is multi-coloured and rolled against a plain floor surface.

(2) The path of a bounced ball is much easier to predict than that of a ball in flight. Athetoid and ataxic children find a bouncing ball easier to catch because the head can remain in the same relative position throughout the performance and the hands can remain in view as well as the ball!

(3) Catching a small ball requires accurate monitoring of its flight and correct manipulation and placement of the hands. There is only a small margin of error between success and failure. A large ball, however, produces more of a gross perceptuo-motor task, with the arms being used to pull the ball into the body. Using large balls, severely handicapped quadriplegic children can be taught to catch.

As a result of such simplification and modification, children progressively learn the basic skills of ball games, until they are eventually able to participate with others in team games. The programme of learning ball skills follows the same sort of pattern as that used in normal Infant Schools.

As suggested earlier, when children are given the opportunity to be successful, they do learn games skills. In turn, participation in team games provides the motivation to produce tremendous ranges of movement in handicapped children, whether they are in wheel-chairs or crawling around on the floor.

CHAPTER SIXTEEN

Learning through Bodily Experience

VERONICA SHERBORNE

The children with whom I work usually function at the level of a normal child aged between two and four years; although some, in special-care classes and in ward classes, function at an even younger level.

I find I can help retarded children in two ways; in relation to their bodies, and in relation to their energy. By increasing the child's awareness of his body, his sense of identity is strengthened, and by learning to experience and direct his energy, the child is helped to focus his attention and to concentrate.

All activities are best experienced and taught through play, and the learning must be enjoyable.

The range of ability in a class of severely retarded children is very wide, but they all have in common the need to find a foundation of security in their own bodies. The early experience of the young baby, which, I feel, is particularly significant, is the experience of his own weight. He senses his body against the ground, his mother, or whatever surface is supporting him. Activities such as rolling, spinning, bouncing, swinging and rocking help the child to experience his weight, and emphasise the wholeness of his body. While these activities are discovered and enjoyed by the normal child, either alone or with the help of a parent, the retarded child needs continual re-inforcement of these early whole-body experiences.

When a child rolls on the floor, he may be thought to express two kinds of commitment. Initially, in allowing his body to rest on the ground, he is accepting the pull of gravity; and when he starts to roll or spin, he gives himself equally to the forces inherent in movement. A confident child will enjoy both, and allow both; but an anxious child will not, for instance, let his head rest on the floor, nor will he enjoy being swung. The most hyperactive and disturbed children will not commit their weight to the ground. Thus the degree to which any child will commit his body is an indication of his self-confidence and self-trust.

I encourage children to move on the ground as if it were water. To this end, it is an essential part of the education that they have the opportunity to play in a swimming-bath regularly.

Having introduced the notion of the body as a whole, I then work on the individual parts. When supported by the floor in rolling, wriggling and a lizard-like crawling, the retarded child is much more aware of the centre of his body (back, shoulders, hips, stomach and chest), than when he is standing up. It is also important for him to experience curling up; for the child who can curl up is secure with himself, and is aware enough of his body to pull all the parts close together so that they are in contact.

164

The sense of touch is very useful in teaching awareness of knees, elbows, hands and face. Hammering with fists on the knees, for example, patting the knees, holding them while they bend and extend, or while walking or jumping, gives the child an increased sensation of the hardness and movement of this part of his anatomy.

The opposite body attitude to that of allowing the body to fall, roll and swing is that of firmness, strength and resistance to outside forces. The baby's first strong pull is the reflex grasp of his hands, while his first strong push is against gravity, in order to crawl. A child experiences his strength best in opposition to something, and an adult provides the best resistance, because he can regulate it so that the child can be successful in his efforts, and yet have to exert all his strength. The children I work with vary enormously in the way they relate to their energy. While some are apathetic and some withdrawn, others are aggressive, and others again are hyperactive.

Most children enjoy sitting back to back and pushing against each other; they enjoy pulling a partner along the floor; they enjoy making an immovable 'rock' using hands, knees and feet to grip the floor, so that they cannot be moved when tested. Some retarded children are able to put hands on each others' shoulders and push. They may tug each other. An important reason for encouraging strength is that a strong, direct movement involves concentration and, however brief this may be, it is essential to help the retarded child to focus his attention. We need to help the child relate to his strength, to organise it, to experience it, to control it. Some children will express strength in tugging but they will not push, because, I believe, they find pushing too much of an involvement with another person. The feeling of strength and stability comes from control of the weight-bearing legs and hips, and by increasing strength and stability we help the child psychologically to be more stable and more sure of himself. There is a playful exchange in the pulling or pushing against someone, and children have a sense of satisfaction and well-being afterwards; they are less likely to be aggressive and spiteful. When children have experienced strength in different ways, they are ready to be sensitive and caring in relation to others.

It is relatively easy to train retarded children in patterns of movement which look, and feel, mechanical. It is extremely difficult to help the retarded child to relate to his own body and to become aware of his energy and the appropriate use of it. On the whole children are attracted to objects outside themselves and never, as it were, 'listen' to themselves. The normal child, first unconsciously and then consciously, responds to information coming from his body, but the retarded child needs continuous help in experiencing his body in many different ways if he is to build up some sense of his identity. Movements which are forceful and movements which are sensitive are expressive of attitudes of mind: a strong statue is a statement 'Here I am'. Self-assertion is as necessary as compassion. The retarded child should extend his experience of 'against' people and 'with' people, against gravity and with gravity, in order to discover himself and begin to develop his potential.

This abbreviated version of Mrs. Sherborne's paper cannot adequately portray the sensitive, practical work she carries out with severely retarded children and many will wish to see her film 'In Touch' (Movement for Mentally Handicapped Children), available from Concord Films, Nacton, Ipswich.

K. S. Holt

CHAPTER SEVENTEEN

Stimulation of Movement:
A Review of Therapeutic Techniques

SOPHIE LEVITT

There are many schools of thought and systems of treatment for the stimulation of movement. This brief review of the most well-known treatment systems attempts to show the essential features of each treatment approach without including all vital details. It is not intended to show how to treat a child with developmental movement problems, but to show the many possibilities for stimulation of movement which are available today.

W. M. Phelps was one of the first to write about therapeutic techniques for handicapped children. Quite soon after Phelps there came Temple-Fay, Eirene Colles, Dr. and Mrs. Bobath, Hermann Kabat, and M. Knott and M. Rood. More recently we have learnt of the work that has been going on for many years in Prague and Budapest by Vojta and Petö respectively. There are many other experts in this field: the ones selected are those whose work is best known.

W. M. Phelps

In the 1940s Dr. Phelps, an orthopaedic surgeon in Baltimore, USA, encouraged physiotherapists, occupational therapists and speech therapists to form themselves into teams to treat cerebral palsied children. The main points of his treatment programme were as follows.

(1) A specific diagnostic classification of the cerebral palsied child was the basis for specific treatment techniques. This included five types of cerebral palsy and many sub-classifications.

(2) A list of fifteen 'modalities' or methods were taught to therapists. These consisted of massage, passive motion, active assisted motion, active motion, resisted motion, rest, conditioned motion, confused motion, combined motion, balance, reach and grasp, skills, relaxation, movement from relaxation and reciprocation.

(3) Braces or calipers were specially designed and developed by Phelps. He prescribed braces to correct deformity and braces to control athetosis.

(4) Equipment for daily living. Many aids for dressing, washing and feeding, and for sitting and locomotion were developed.

(5) Muscle education for spastics and training in joint control for athetoids was the emphasis of the largely orthopaedic view of cerebral palsy. Motor development was rarely discussed as a foundation for therapy.

Muscle education for spastics was also developed in specific ways by a number of other cerebral palsy authorities such as Pohl in America and Plum in Denmark and many orthopaedic therapists and doctors in Britain.

Although many people today dismiss Phelps' approach, there is much of interest which we can still use for our patients. Braces (calipers) are needed by some children, although they need not be as extensive or used for as many years as Phelps recommended. Muscle education is necessary before and after orthopaedic surgery. Many of the aids devised at Phelps' clinic form the basis of occupational therapy today.

Temple-Fay

Temple-Fay was working in Philadelphia at about the same time as Phelps. He was a neurosurgeon and differed from Phelps in his view of cerebral palsy and mentally subnormal children. His main points can be summarised as follows.

(1) Movement patterns, rather than muscle education, were the foundations for therapeutic techniques.

(2) *Phylogenetic* movement patterns were recommended as these were patterns that were seen in simple nervous systems in the animal kingdom. He encouraged treatment by saying that, although there was an incurable brain lesion, primitive movement patterns still remained in the medulla, pons, and mid-brain and could produce activity. He devised progressive movement patterns which started with primitive levels of squirming, or head and trunk rolling, followed by primitive creeping in a homolateral pattern with upper and lower limb moving on the same side and then followed by the contralateral pattern when the arm moved on the opposite side to the leg. After creeping, the child was trained to crawl and then go on hands and feet in the 'bear walk' and finally trained to walk upright. He compared these levels of development to patterns seen in the lower animals such as amphibians, then four-footed mammals, and finally in man.

(3) A strict sequence of phylogenetic development was stressed.

(4) The children were taught the progressive movement patterns by passive motion and then encouraged to carry them out actively.

(5) No braces and no other exercises were used. Reflex movements were employed to strengthen muscles, and to relax spasticity.

There is much that is controversial in this system just as there is in any system. Doman and Delacato are using most of Fay's methods in their approach, but seem to be making many more demands on parents to 'pattern' their handicapped child than was done when I was at Fay's clinic. I also find that passive patterning is not as helpful in training movement as other methods. However, creeping is valuable in treating many children, if it is used within a total perspective of child development. I have also found the omission of adequate training of posture and balance reactions untenable.

H. Kabat and M. Knott

Kabat and Knott in California devised the treatment system called 'proprioceptive neuromuscular facilitation'. Kabat is no longer working there, but Margaret Knott, Dorothy Voss and others are still teaching and using these methods. The main ideas in this treatment approach are as follows.

(1) Movement patterns rather than muscle education of individual muscle groups are recommended. However, the movement patterns taught should be those used by man in such functions as rolling over, getting up, locomotion and various daily skills using the upper limb.

(2) The diagonal and rotatory aspects of movement patterns were observed by Kabat. Every movement pattern used in the therapeutic techniques has a diagonal direction. Rotation and flexion-extension and abduction or adduction are the elements of the patterns.

(3) Sensory afferent stimuli were shown to stimulate motion. Proprioception is emphasised although the techniques include touch, auditory and visual stimuli as well as the stimuli from stretch, pressure, and muscle contraction.

(4) Resistance is used to facilitate stronger muscle action within the synergic patterns of movement. Various methods are used to adjust the degree of resistance. It is also important to know where to apply resistance to get a local effect or an effect in another part of the body associated with the movement pattern.

(5) Ice treatments are used to relax or inhibit hypertonus. Relaxation techniques of a special kind are also included for selected cases.

These methods are useful in many cerebral palsied children, are particularly good for weakness in any condition, and can be used to train motor skills. Although not mentioned by most authorities writing about proprioceptive neuro-muscular facilitation, I have found that modifications should be made when treating the various types of cerebral palsy.

Margaret Rood

Before leaving the American scene, it is important to mention the well-known authority on movement stimulation, Margaret Rood, who is both a physiotherapist and an occupational therapist. Her approach is based on many neurophysiological experiments. The theories are highly controversial. She stresses the following aspects.

(1) Afferent stimuli to facilitate and inhibit movement.

(2) Classification of different muscle work and sensory impulses in relation to techniques.

(3) An ontogenetic skeletal development sequence is used as a developmental set of milestones which she follows dogmatically.

(4) Reflexes of many kinds are used to stimulate movement and muscle actions at an unconscious or involuntary level.

Karl and Berta Bobath

These authorities have developed their treatment techniques over twenty years or more. Both are well-known in Britain and their main ideas are as follows.

(1) The main difficulty is over-action of tonic reflex activity. These tonic reflexes must be assessed in each patient and 'reflex inhibitory movement patterns' used to counteract them.

(2) A developmental sequence is followed according to each child.

(3) Primitive reflexes seen in early infancy should be inhibited and more mature neurological reactions facilitated, especially in retarded children who still persist in using these primitive reflexes. Conscious participation is unnecessary in the treatment of babies and children.

(4) All-day management should supplement treatment sessions. In fact, correct management involves treatment. Nancy Finnie (1968) gives advice to parents on methods of handling and equipment in her book entitled 'Handling the Cerebral Palsied Child at Home'.

Eirene Colles

Eirene Colles was a British pioneer of cerebral palsy treatment. She stressed neuromotor development as a basis for treatment. Her developmental milestones were dogmatically presented. She also considered it important to plan the whole day of the child and not rely solely on short physiotherapy sessions. Colles suggested that there should be cerebral palsy therapists rather than combinations of physiotherapists, occupational therapists and speech therapists. She thought this would help the child to have a more successful total therapeutic day, and also counteract the separation of the different professional disciplines.

V. Vojta

Vojta worked in Czechoslovakia for about twenty years before moving to Cologne, Germany, where he now works. His approach is based on Temple-Fay and Kabat, and also on many of his own ideas. His methods consist primarily of the following.

(1) Reflex creeping. Creeping patterns are facilitated by various 'trigger' points and afferent stimuli of touch, stretch and pressure.

(2) Resistance is also used in order to facilitate a stronger movement or reflex response. If the child can augment his motion by conscious participation, this is also utilised in treatment. However, this conscious participation is not essential and so it is possible to treat babies from birth onwards.

(3) Reflex rolling techniques are used to provoke turning over and rising. Rising reflexes are also stimulated within the creeping complex.

(4) Movement patterns are recommended. Vojta analysed the muscle actions of the creeping complex, of reflex rolling and of other movements used by normal babies. Physiotherapists stimulate movement patterns using these muscle groups and avoid provoking 'pathological' reactions and movements.

Vojta, Bobath, Colles and many others strongly recommend early treatment. Vojta uses a detailed list of reflexes as an aid in the examination of the baby in order to decide whether treatment is indicated or not, and also at what developmental level treatment should be commenced.

Petö

Professor Petö of Budapest devised a system of treatment which integrates therapy with education. His main recommendations were as follows.

(1) Conductors should be specially trained to treat handicapped children. The

conductor integrates treatment and education, using principles of learning.
(2) The children are treated in groups.
(3) The training involves an all-day programme.
(4) Rhythmic intention is the technique used for training movement. The children state the intended motion and then carry it out to the rhythm of counting or an operative word repeated during motion.
(5) Movements are devised in such a way that they are the elements of a task or motor skill. The child is taught the purpose of each movement. The movements are repeated in various contexts within a carefully-planned day.
(6) Individual treatment sessions may be used for some children to help them participate more adequately in their group.

Conclusion

Therapists treating children today are fortunate in being able to develop a repertoire of many different techniques for stimulating movement. They must have a good assessment of each child in order to select the most appropriate methods of treatment for each individual. Many of the theories upon which treatment systems are based are controversial. As it is difficult to prove which approach is superior to any of the others, it is suggested that an eclectic approach is desirable, and the treatment planned to match the needs of the child.

BIBLIOGRAPHY

American Journal of Physical Medicine (1967) *An Exploratory and Analytical Survey of Therapeutic Exercise. American Journal of Physical Medicine,* vol. 26. Baltimore: Williams and Wilkins.
Bobath, B. (1963) 'Treatment principles and planning in cerebral palsy.' *Physiotherapy,* **49**, 122.
—— (1965) *Abnormal Postural Reflex Activity Caused by Brain Lesions.* London: Heinemann.
—— (1971) 'Motor development, its effect on general development, and application to the treatment of cerebral palsy.' *Physiotherapy,* **57**, 526.
Bobath, K. (1966) *The Motor Deficit in Patients with Cerebral Palsy.* Clinics in Developmental Medicine, no. 23. London: S.I.M.P./Heinemann.
—— (1971) 'The normal postural reflex mechanism and its deviation in children with cerebral palsy.' *Physiotherapy,* **57**, 515.
Cotton, E. (1965) 'The Institute for Movement Therapy and School for "Conductors", Budapest, Hungary.' *Developmental Medicine and Child Neurology,* **7**, 437.
—— (1970) 'Integration of treatment and education in cerebral palsy.' *Physiotherapy,* **56**, 143.
—— Parnwell, M. (1967) 'From Hungary: the Petö Method.' *Special Education,* **56**, 7.
—— —— (1968) 'Conductive education.' *Journal of Mental Subnormality,* **14**, 26.
Decker, R. (1962) *Motor Integration.* Springfield, Ill.: C.C. Thomas.
Egel, P. F. (1948) *Technique of Treatment for the Cerebral Palsy Child.* St. Louis: C. V. Mosby.
Ellis, E. (1967) *Physical Management of Developmental Disorders.* Clinics in Developmental Medicine, no. 26. London: S.I.M.P./Heinemann.
Fay, T (1946) 'Observations on the rehabilitation of movement in cerebral palsy problems.' *West Virginia Medical Journal,* **42**, 77.
—— (1948) 'The neurophysical aspects of therapy in cerebral palsy.' *Archives of Physical Medicine,* **29**, 327.
Finnie, N. R. (1968) *Handling the Young Cerebral Palsied Child at Home.* London: Wm. Heinemann.
Gillette, H. E. (1969) *Systems of Therapy in Cerebral Palsy.* Springfield, Ill.: C. C. Thomas.
Goff, B. (1969) 'Appropriate afferent stimulation.' *Physiotherapy,* **55**, 9.
Knott, M., Voss, D. E. (1968) *Proprioceptive Neuromuscular Facilitation,* 2nd ed. New York: Hoeber.
Levitt, S. (1962) *Physiotherapy in Cerebral Palsy.* Springfield, Ill.: C. C. Thomas.
—— (1966) 'Proprioceptive neuromuscular facilitation techniques in cerebral palsy.' *Physiotherapy,* **52**, 46.

—— (1969) 'The treatment of cerebral palsy and Proprioreceptive Neuromuscular Facilitation Techniques. "On the treatment of Spastic Paresis"'. *Sjuk Gymnasten*, **27**, 3.

—— (1970) 'P.N.F. in cerebral palsy.' Proceedings of the World Congress on Physical Therapy, Amsterdam.

Phelps, W. M. (1941) 'The rehabilitation of cerebral palsy.' *Southern Medical Journal*, **34**, 770.

—— (1952) 'The rôle of physical therapy in cerebral palsy.' *In Orthopedic Appliances Atlas I.* Ann Arbor: Edwards.

Sattely, C. (1962) 'Approaches to the treatment of patients with neuromuscular dysfunction.' Study Course VI, *Third International Congress of World Federation of Occupational Therapists.* Iowa: Wm. C. Brown.

Voss, D. E. (1959) 'Proprioceptive neuromuscular facilitation. Application of patterns and techniques in occupational therapy.' *American Journal of Occupational Therapy*, **13**, 191.

Wolf, J. M. (1969) *The Results of Treatment in Cerebral Palsy.* Springfield, Ill.: C. C. Thomas.

CHAPTER EIGHTEEN

Implications of Movement and Child Development for Parents, Therapists, Teachers and Doctors

(Summarised by K. S. Holt from reports by N. Finnie, M. Gilbertson,
G. J. Higgon and K. S. Holt)

The previous chapters reveal the complexity of human movement, the importance of movement in child development, and the need to study the effects of impaired movement upon the development of the disabled child. If the practical implications of these deliberations are understood, more active and realistic actions to help disabled children may follow.

Everyone who attended the original symposium or who read these proceedings afterwards will have made some conclusions relevant to their own interests and needs. It is not possible to represent every range of opinion and interpretation, but it was felt worthwhile to discuss the implications of this report with respect to four specific groups, namely parents, therapists, teachers and doctors. The views expressed at the symposium are summarised in this chapter.

Parents are eager to learn as much as they can about their babies. Although they look for movements (for example when their baby reaches out with his hand, or when he walks), they often do not understand how best they can encourage such movements, nor do they appreciate the variety of activities and experiences which may result from movement. This information can be usefully incorporated into the developmental advice and guidance which should be available to all parents.

In the case of children whose movements are reduced or limited, parents express concern because their children are not performing various activities (*e.g.* walking) at the right times, but they seldom appreciate the wider effects of this restricted movement. They cannot begin to understand all that movement means to their child, nor carry out any form of activity or stimulation with him (or her) until they have overcome their anxieties and fears. Their child is not doing what he should be doing. He is disabled, abnormal, deformed. Added to these anxieties are fears that they might make him worse, and uncertainties because they do not know what to do for the best. Expert guidance from paediatricians and therapists is needed to help parents overcome these fears. Learning about movement and the uses a child makes of movement in the course of development helps parents to overcome their difficulties and restores their confidence to do things with their child—especially activities which involve movement. They can then be taught how to stimulate a child's movements, and how to plan his activities to make his movements purposeful.

Throughout the day, from rising in the morning to going to bed at night, there are many ways a skilled therapist can help parents to respond to, handle, and stimulate their child suffering motor impairment. Despite the magnitude and importance of this work, it is not a substitute for the specific therapy which may be required in some cases. However, specific therapy proves to be more effective and worthwhile in those cases where the daily programme is given full attention.

Therapists clearly need to understand all that has been written about movement and child development. The anxieties of parents with a handicapped child are mentioned above, and it is to therapists that parents turn to get the help and understanding they seek. Sometimes the therapists sympathise but feel they cannot help because they do not themselves appreciate all the facets of movement and child development. These situations arise all too often and illustrate that sympathy without knowledge does not lead to true understanding and help. Although many therapists work with children, they receive very little training in child development. This needs to be put right urgently, and information about the developmental implications of movement should be included in both undergraduate and postgraduate training for therapists.

Another important lesson for therapists from this study is the value of a critical analysis of all one is doing and of accurate recording. All too often an enquiry into the nature and value of therapy is seen as a criticism and is resisted. This inhibits progress. It is to be hoped that the advantages which come from a deeper understanding of any subject will have been revealed in this report and will encourage therapists to analyse and to record their everyday practical work.

Much of every child's life is spent in school and the implications of movement and child development with respect to the school situation deserves special consideration. The school environment provides excellent opportunities for teachers (especially for teachers of physically disabled children) to develop creative motor activity programmes for the children. Such programmes provide both the benefits of stimulation of motor activities and the direction of these activities to purposeful ends. The precise programme depends upon the children's ages and their abilities: whereas play figures prominently in the nursery situation, games are more important for the older children. The intensity of motor activity programmes covers a wide range, from the work of an enlightened teacher who appreciates the relationship between movement and child development and uses this knowledge in the organisation of her class activities, to the intense therapeutic and physical education programmes which are carried out in some cases. Teachers who appreciate the developmental rôle of movement better understand their colleagues' work in therapy and physical education and this leads to closer teamwork between the members of the related disciplines.

Once paediatricians realise the significance of movement in relation to child development, they recognise the narrowness of their earlier concepts of child disability, the scope of developmentally orientated therapy for those suffering motor disabilities, and the importance of studying in depth the neurophysiological basis of development and therapy. This is a major reorientation of attitudes and practice. The tradition that diagnosis (*i.e.* identifying and labelling) is the all-important peak of the medical exercise does not apply in the case of disabled children. Interpretation of the developmental implications of the child's disability is essential in this work because it leads to a fuller understanding of the children's problems and provides a sound basis for planning their treatment and care. These features are well illustrated in this collection of symposium papers. As with the other professions, as doctors realise the importance of movement, they are able to give more effective advice, they come to understand the work of others, and they more readily and easily work together with the other team members.

Name Index

Diamond, M. C.; **29.**
Dierfu, W.; **144.**
Dimitrijevič, M. R.; 45, **48.**
Dixon, K.; 139, **143.**
Douglas; V.; **144.**
Drillien, C. M.; 14, **17.**

E

Egel, P. F.; **170.**
Eisenberg, L.; 15, **17.**
Eklund, G.; **48.**
Eldred, E.; 25, **30.**
Elliott, J.; 103, **110.**
Ellis, E.; **170.**
Evarts, E. V.; 38, 42, **48,** 106, **110.**
Euler, C. von; **48.**

F

Fay, T.; 166, 167, 169, **170.**
Finnie, N. R.; **170.**
Fitzgerald, J. E.; 22, **33.**
Foerster, O.; 45, **49.**
Fog, E.; 111, **118.**
Fog, M.; 111, **118.**
Freeman, L. W.; 45, **49.**
Freidin, M. R.; **18.**
Fulton, J. F.; 26, **31.**

G

Galambos, R.; 28, **30.**
Gamper, E.; 26, **30.**
Gardner, E.; 28, **30.**
Gassell, M. M.; 45, **49.**
Gaze, R. M.; 28, **30.**
Gesell, A.; 20, 22, 23, 25, 26, **30.**
Gidoni, E. A.; 128, **131.**
Gillette, H. E.; **170.**
Goff, B.; **170.**
Goldiamond, I.; 142, **144.**
Goldie, L.; 29.
Goodenough, F. L.; 111, **118.**
Gooddy, W.; 20, **30.**
Graham, P.; 11, **13,** 32, **144.**
Granit, R.; 25, 26, 28, 29, **30,** 41, **49.**
Grant, E. C.; 134, **143.**
Grant, Q. R.; 134, **143.**
Greenberg, L.; 14, **17.**
Greene, P. H.; 108, **110.**

H

Hagbarth, K. -E.; 28, **30, 31.**
Hamilton, W. J.; 20, 22, 23, 24, 26, **30.**
Hammond, P. H.; 42, **49.**
Hare, C. C.; 28, **31.**

Harrison, A.; 47, **49,** 59, 66, 68, **74,** 75, 85, 96, **101,** 104, **110.**
Hastings, M. L.; **118.**
Hefferline, R. F.; 40, **49,** 104, **110.**
Heimburger, R. F.; 45, **49.**
Hein, A.; 105; **110.**
Held, R.; 10, **13,** 25, **31,** 38, 39, **49,** 105, **110.**
Hernández-Peón, R.; 26, 28, **31.**
Hewer, E. E.; 23 **31.**
Hines, M.; 26, **31.**
Hodgkins, J.; 24, **31.**
Hogg, I. D.; 22, **31.**
Holland, P.; **143.**
Holst, E. von; 38, **50,** 105, **110.**
Holt, K. S.; 119, **123.**
Hooker, D.; 20, 22, 23, 25, 28, **31.**
Hopkins, I. J.; 29.
Hornbeim, T. F.; **49.**
Horton, M.; 145.
Hromada, J.; 24, **31.**
Hudson, B. W.; **17, 143.**
Humphrey, T.; 22, 23, 24, 25, 26, **31.**
Hunt, R. S.; **49.**
Hutt, C.; 119, **123.**
Hutt, S. J.; **123.**

I

Iggo, A.; 25, **31.**
Ingram, T. T. S.; 14, **17.**

J

Jackson, J. H.; 38, **49.**
Jacobs, M. J.; 22, **31.**
Jansen, J. K. S.; 45, **49.**
Jones, B.; 4, **7.**
Jones, H. E.; 112, **118.**
Jones, R.; **144.**

K

Kabat, H.; 166, 167, 168.
Kagan, J.; 16, **17.**
Karpovich, P. V.; 35, **49.**
Kastenbaum, R.; 146, 156.
Keech, D.; **29.**
Kember, P. A.; 129, **131.**
Kennard, M. A.; 26, **31.**
Kenny, T. J.; 14, **17,** 133, **143.**
Kenshalo, D. R.; 24, 28, **31.**
Kingsbury, B. F.; 22, 25, **31.**
Klein, D. A.; **118.**
Knight, J.; 25, **32.**
Knobloch, H.; 14, **18.**
Knott, M.; 166, 167, **170.**
Ko, W. H.; 139, **143.**

177

Subject Index

Muscle contraction, 35
    eccentric, 117
    isometric, 117
    isotonic, 117
Muscle tension, cues to, 56
Music, 157
Myelinisation, 23

N

Neurological maturation, 9

O

Object permanence, 149
Observational techniques, 112, 119, 132

P

Parkinson's disease, 75
Perceptual development, 10
Performance, consistency of, 116
Personality deviations, 133
Peto, Professor, 169
Phelps, W. M., 166
Physical disability, effects of, 146
Physical education, 162
Physical skills, 8, 12
Physiotherapist, 10
Pincer grasp, 149
Play, 164
Posture,
    adjustment, 19
    anti-gravity, 2
    controlled, 47
    in spastic persons, 46
Procaine, 45
Proprioceptive neuromuscular facilitation, 168
Pyramidal tract, 42

R

Reach, 148
Reaching, visually directed, 5, 107
Reaction, chain, 2
Reflex,
    abnormal, 46, 75
    activity, 35
    asymmetrical tonic neck, 2
    basis of early neuromuscular behaviour, 25
    cervical arthrokinetic, 24
    clasp-knife, 47
    creeping, 169
    grasp, 2
    'H', 45

    hyper, 46
    Moro, 2, 46
    polysynaptic, 22
    primitive, 46, 75, 169
    stretch, 37, 42
    times, 24
Relaxation, 76
Release, 149
Response,
    conscious, 157
    speed of, 111
    to music, 157
Retarded children, 164
Rhythmic intention, 170
Rood, M., 168
Rotary pursuit, 111

S

Sensorimotor integration, 4
Sensory information, 38
Signal detection theory, 58
Skill, 102
    components of, 117
    defined, 9, 116
    development of, 102, 106
    of handicapped child, 162
Social development, 11
Sollwert, 105
Spastic individuals, 51, 52, 75, 78, 81, 84, 91
Spastic syndrome, 45
Specific learning difficulties, 133
Speech difficulties, 161
Spina bifida, 9, 145
Sub routines, 43, 103, 106

T

Tactile exploration, 5
Teacher, 162
Team games, 163
Temple-Fay, 167
Tempo, 158
Tendon jerk, 37
Therapist, 160, 173
Therapy, 12, 166
Transfer, 148

U

Unidextrous approach, 148
Upper limb function, 145

181